To Pat

Shine On Light

Sandra M Prusher

AWESOMENESS CUBED PRAYER WARRIORING

*From the Heart of a Healer, Holistic Vet,
and Single Mom*

SANDRA M. SNELL, DVM, CVA, PSC. D

BALBOA.
PRESS
A DIVISION OF HAY HOUSE

Balboa Press books may be ordered through booksellers or by contacting:

Balboa Press
A Division of Hay House
1663 Liberty Drive
Bloomington, IN 47403
www.balboapress.com
1 (877) 407-4847

Print information available on the last page.

ISBN: 978-1-9822-1493-7 (sc)
ISBN: 978-1-9822-1495-1 (hc)
ISBN: 978-1-9822-1494-4 (e)

Library of Congress Control Number: 2018912937

Balboa Press rev. date: 11/16/2018

Contents

Testimonials

4/20/18

Since I personally have decided to follow an holistic approach to my health care, it made sense to do the same for my dogs. I was not happy with a local Veterinarian for quite some time so I decided to try Doctor Sandy after hearing many positive comments about her. I was not disappointed, as soon as I entered the Sycamore Animal Hospital with my beagle named Bobbi, a calming effect washed over me. I felt comfortable and more importantly, Bobbi felt comfortable.

Bobbi's first session with Sandy was so neat, after being worked on for her congestive heart failure, Bobbi yawned a few times and took a little nap, totally relaxed and content. To witness what had just happened was truly eye opening into how the holistic sessions work. Sandy was in total sync to what was happening with Bobbi and what pain she was having. It certainly was not a normal visit to the Vet, and I am so happy it was not. Sandy does not rush through anything, she gets to know the dog and then a plan is mapped out for the best results. Sandy loves what she is doing and it is very evident when talking to her.

Sandy was able to give Bobbi an extra year and a half that conventional medicine could not, I am grateful for that, but wish I had found her before Bobbi was diagnosed with congestive heart failure. If both of my dogs had Sandy for a Vet from the puppy stage on, many problems we encountered throughout their lifetimes could have been prevented. Bobbi and my collie named Carmen, ended up living to 15 and 16 years respectfully, because of Sandy. Thank you Doctor Sandy Snell for your knowledge and for caring so much about pets and people, you have a special gift from our Lord.

Joe Kramer

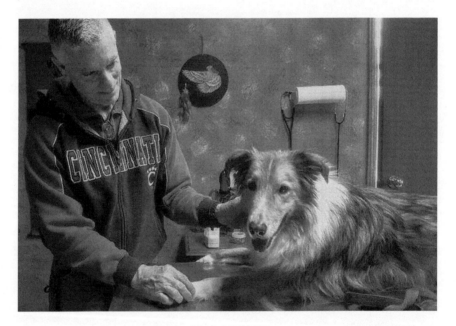

5/7/18

My exposure to Dr. Snell and all of her energy methods for healing, clearing, and cleaning for both people and pets had felt very much like something out of the Wizard of Oz. Like a Kansas tornado, I was swept away from the gray world of physical, mental, emotional, energetic and spiritual issues and found the colorful version of myself by receiving her treatments and by applying what resonated with me from her "velvet wizards bag" of self help techniques. While everyone's journey along their yellow brick road is unique to them, the tools and techniques given in this book can help us all navigate our way back home with a little more brains, a little more courage, and a little more heart. I am grateful for all the ways Dr. Snell has taught and reminded me to click my ruby red shoes.....

W.Darling
YALMTYK

6/10/18

I met Dr. Sandy Snell in 2009 when my 18 year old beloved pony (Tony) was severely foundered. Tony could barely stand and walking was very difficult for him. I had 3 different veterinarians tell me there was no treatment and no hope and that I needed to euthanize my little buddy asap.

I searched the internet for a Holistic Veterinarian in Ohio and found Dr. Snell. I called her at 6pm and told her about my ponies condition. Even though I lived an hour and a half away and she had never met me, she jumped in her van and came straight to my barn.

Dr. Snell worked on Tony for at least two hours using multiple therapies including Chiropractic, Reiki, and Energy Healing. When she was done, Tony could move freely and was trotting around the arena.

Tony lived three more years.

Dr. Snell has helped restore my health and has helped my numerous horses, dogs, and cats. Dr. Snell has shown me and taught me the incredible power of energy and distance healing.

Ruth Kaplan

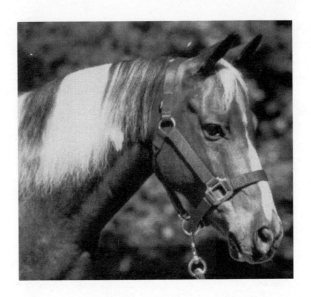

6/12/18

"Throughout the years of knowing Dr. Snell she has helped many of my horses. For example I had a horse that had a fear of people and was very painful in the back; she worked on him and we saw an immediate response for him. He was more relaxed and could be ridden without having discomfort. While working on my horses she has you feel the before and after she adjusts them and there is always a big difference. Dr. Snell has always made the horse she has worked on for me ten times better than before."

Odessa Harrington

6/19/18

This testimonial took me a long time to start because I didn't know where to even begin. There is something about Sandy that is special, simple and pure. Its the worlds mysteries that make us question "why?" and then realize it was just meant to be. The earths energies shifting and our personal energies given to the universe brought us together. I am forever grateful to just know she is there when I need her. She's there to take any problem I have with myself, family or animals and devotes her whole self to helping others. The only thing I would change would be moving her next to me so I could see her and absorb her energy everyday.

Kati Christner

Sandy has helped all my animals and my family soooooo much through the years that I have known her. I don't know what I would do without her. Love you sooo much 😎 ☐

Barb Oberhaus

6/20/18

When we brought Ryley to Dr. Snell he had hurt his back and had a bulging disc and could not stand up because his rear legs would not work. After 2 hours of her working on him, he was able to walk out of Sycamore Animal Hospital. He kept getting stronger with each treatment. It's only been one year and he is going for walks everyday with no problems. We are forever grateful for her and could not thank Dr. Snell enough ☐☐☐

Becky Winner

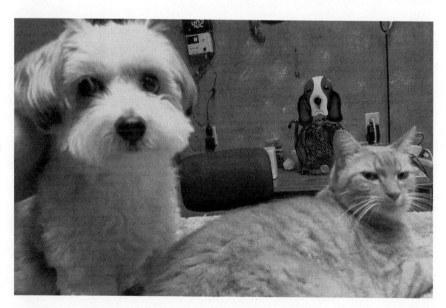

I have been going to Dr. Snell for many years and I have had her work on me and my dogs. I can honestly say with each visit you don't know what to expect but you and your dog will be in a better place when you leave. Many thanks to her and her staff.

Robin Ford of "Marks Agility Equipment" and Robin Ford Dog Training.

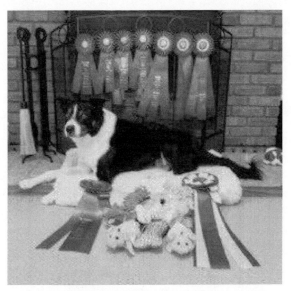

Norwoods Biggest Rival Elite Nose Work,
XF,MXJ,MX,HSAs,RAE,CDX

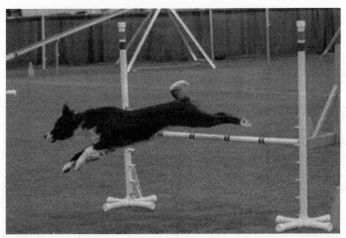

Norwoods Good Karma ORT B/A/C MX,MXJ,OF,HSAS

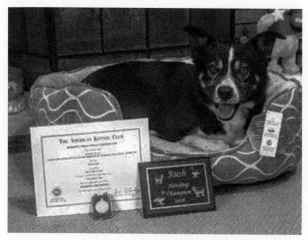

HC, MACH Norwoods Good Feeling Elite Nose
Work, MJB,MB,XF,HXAds,HXBd

6/28/18

I really don't remember how I found out about Sandra Snell, but I'm so glad I got to bring her into my life.

One if my first encounters with Sandra's amazing special talents, was with my beloved GSD, Harley. He had the dreaded "itchies". I tried everything, drugs, shots, shave the spot and treat with anything. Nothing worked, it was driving my baby crazy and hurt him. So, to Sandra off we go, with all the samples she asked for. During the visit, I watched her n him carefully, thinking, how is this going to work? After all, I have been to two Vets n tried everything....right!? No, not everything. It was a blessing, she said get him home and leave him in side for the evening. I did. I was amazed, this dog crashed on the floor, in a dead sleep. I actually tapped him a few times to make sure he was alive....lol. The next morning he was so happy and feeling great. I watched the hot spot, which was infected when I took him to her, heal. It just went away, he never itched again. I never treated him, didn't change his food or anything.

My beloved Harley passed at the age of 12 years. Happy and healthy. Thanks to Sandra.

But that wasn't the end, she treated my next GSD/Lab, also for the same thing. This time Sandra was my first trip for Zachary. And the results were amazing. No drugs, just Sandra's special touch.

Traci Lord

7/22/18

"Dr Sandra Snell is THE most amazing Vet/Human that I have ever met. She heals minds, souls, spirits as well as our bodies. Her Holistic method of treatment has been spot-on with many of my various dogs as well as myself. Thank you Universe for guiding her to us ☮ □."

Debra Garner

7/22/18

In today's day and age it's hard to come by a person who is intuitive and knows how to engage and express their gifts. Being in the field of compassion and skill, it's easy to become confident in taught skill and lose faith in your given skill. The best thing that has happened to me in my short time in my career was meeting Dr. Sandy Snell – someone who has mastered the art of blending taught and given skill. I met Sandy in December 2013 after I cold-called her for veterinary shadowing experience. I'll never forget she said "come on a Wednesday night and make sure you like us first." Long story short, I did like the whole family at Sycamore Animal Hospital (SAH), a lot, and spent lots of time with them through the rest of my undergraduate career.

From a professional perspective, Sandy taught me many things – chiropractic, oils, acu-techniques, and more. I spent hours pouring over "Modern Essentials," observing adjustments, working on pets. We had car rides to discuss theories and ideas, lunch breaks to laugh and enjoy each other's presence. I got to know and enjoy Sandy's daughter and staff. The four of us had many afternoons in the office eating pizza and sharing stories and smiles, but also teaching each other aroma touch, reiki and much more. Those afternoons kept me sane through undergrad, and definitely kept me in order!

Spending time at SAH taught me life lessons I have taken from then to now, mainly to take care of myself and make time for what I love. Sandy taught me some of the most valuable lessons of healing that I have, and will continue to carry through vet school, which is to keep an open mind and the power of positive healing. I have spent a lot of time considering the place and use of modern and traditional medicine, and I have a lot to thank Sandy for, in terms of my appreciation for either approach. Without my time at SAH I doubt I would be half of who I am now, and I certainly know Sandy has had a huge impact on the person I am continuing to grow into today. Thank you for all you do and have done, Sandy!!

Vicky Johnson, BS
Ohio State University
College of Veterinary Medicine
Class of 2020

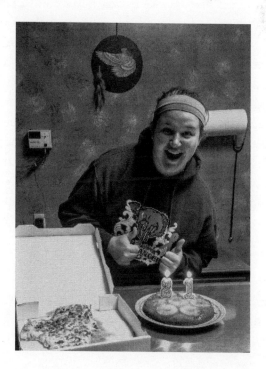

7/24/18

Doctor Snell how can you describe her besides amazing.
Always there for my animals.
Not only has she held my hand when we have lost my fur babies.
She has been a mentor and inspiration to my teaching and healing!

Laura Freeman

8/6/18

Dr. Snell has mended and helped many horses at Lane Of Dreams Farm LLC.

One appointment with a particular horse sold me forever on her powers of healing …. not just physical but spiritually helping this horse be a happy, contributing member of our farms lesson program.

"Chief" is a black and white paint gelding that was given to us. Right from the start, Chief seemed like he was never comfortable in his own skin. He would worry in a stall and try to escape to the point of breaking door latches but then try to get back into the barn. It made no sense and he was very hard to manage. We tried putting him out with the herd, which they DID NOT like him at all! The other horses didn't even want to stand near him and always ran him away. He wasn't comfortable in cross ties and would not stand still when single tied either. We tried tying in the isle, in the wash stall, in regular stalls and he just could not stand still. He acted like something was constantly "after him". After over 25 years of horse experience, I was at my wits end with this horse since riding him came with the same results. He just could not focus on what a rider was asking, for fear something was going to get him and I could not figure out how to help him!

It made me so sad because I truly believed that he was given to us for reason…which was to be a lesson horse that was given a second chance to be happy and loved.

I had seen Sandy in the previous years for many different reasons.... horse and personal. I had struggled with my back & Sandy always helped alleviate the pain and eventually cured it. She helped clear my mind as well and be spiritually healthy. When she came to work on the horses, I found it fascinating her healing ways and she always encouraged me to expand my abilities to learn the healing ways too! I think she felt that I had the gift and my mind was open to trying it. I told Sandy that I was raised Catholic and worried about the good and BAD in the world and that I feared that I would not be educated enough to protect myself or loved ones had the BAD reared its ugly head. To many horror movies, I guess???

Now back to Chief....when it was his turn to see Sandy... I brought the little paint thru the stall door and into the isle where Sandy stood... Sandy gave a big sigh...quickly sat down....looked like she was going to vomit...and said to me...."Julie, remember your biggest fear??? Well,here it is!" She was quiet for a long time while she put her hands all over this horse and the more she touched him the more he wiggled and jigged and danced. She quickly put together a shell of burning sage which we fanned the smoke all around Chief and to my surprise he quickly settled down and seemed to enjoy the ritual. While I started to get the feeling that we were" summoning evil" and it WAS NOT HAPPY AT All!! The hair on my arm started to stand up and I felt the dark presence getting madder and madder that we were trying to free this poor beast of its evil hold on him! We prayed. Sandy broke out the salt and began to make the star of David on the ground around the horse, on his forehead and body to try to release him from the attachment. She encouraged me to do the same and at one point ....Sandy told me to sprinkle salt on anything that I wanted to protect as the attachment was losing grip and was looking for someone or something else to attach too! I ran to the barn cats, other horses,other people in the barn which included my daughter, sprinkled the salt and prayed. She also said to pray over anyone that I loved to protect them as well, even if they weren't here.

The barn seemed to get darker and darker. I could almost see the dark shadow looming on the edge of the property, hiding, waiting to attach to something else. I could feel the entities anger and then ….then… suddenly it became lighter, I could open my eyes wider to let the light in. I could breathe easier and felt free. The feeling of hopelessness and evil was gone, replaced with love, light, and warmth.

The feelings of pure evil and hate that I experienced that day still make my hair on the back of my neck stand up. The sense of urgency to protect the ones that I love from the unspeakable evil was overwhelming. As we concluded the cleansing session with Chief (who at this point is standing totally still with his head down, exhausted) Our task was a success(scary as it was!!!) and to this day…Mr. Chief is still works at Lane Of Dreams Farm as a happy lesson horse and gets along with all the horses! He has helped many a student look inside themselves to find the real reasons for personal struggles. It had nothing to do with horse training and so glad that Chief being labeled a "naughty" horse was then able to be cured by Dr. Sandy Snell.

Julie Vogel

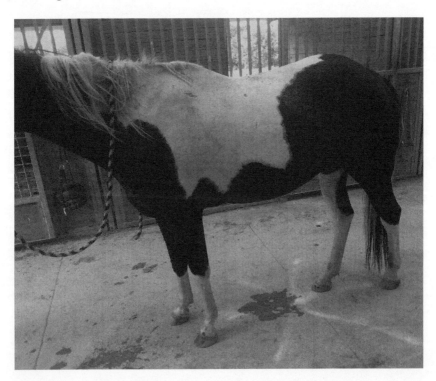

APRIL AND SUSAN'S STORY

April is a declawed cat that I rescued from a bad situation. She likes to be up high which is not a good thing for a cat with no front claws. Because of this she has had a number of bad falls. She started having seizures and was not able to walk very well. I took her to Dr Sandy Snell, who worked with April to realign your spine and to help her with the pain. April had several treatments and her seizures have stopped. She is now able to walk again without pain. Dr Sandy has given her a better lease on life.

April is not the only one who has benefit from Dr. Sandy numerous skills. I suffer from kidney stones. I have had to go to ER multiple times from being in so much pain. I have have an MRI done and it found 7 stones on the right side and 4 to 5 on left. My doctor said not to worry about them unless they were moving. Dr. Sandy did Reiki and Aromatouch Techniques and it was very relaxing and it made the pain slide away. I was better able to do my job with lot less pain.

Later, I injured my right knee and was in a lot of pain and unable to walk well. I was sent to a specialist who only made the pain worse. I made an appointment with Dr Sandy and she worked on me it was painless and very relaxing. I had several treatments and was able to start walking again without hardly any discomfort.

I'm so glad our paths have crossed.

Namaste
Susan Senn Coleman

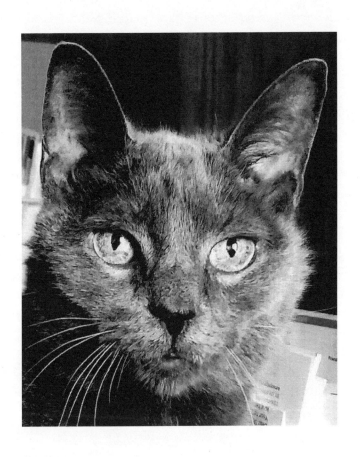

PART OF THE MOTTER CREWS STORY

Doc

My family has always been animal lovers. Currently, mainly due to our kids, we seem to have more pets than most. One of our rescues is Doc, a senior Australian Shepherd. We fell in love with this breed a while ago, and when one of our Aussie mix dogs died of old age our daughter decided she wanted another Aussie. She got approved by an Aussie rescue group and they brought two dogs for us to pick from. She liked the younger, mix color that looked a little like the dog she lost. The other dog is a blue merle named Doc. Doc was six at the time. He also was a bit shy and had a goofy haircut. We kind of felt sorry for this older dog that no one seemed to want. So, we took him.

Doc is a very sweet dog, and, oh, is he ball crazy he loves to chase balls. We invented a game called Doc keep away where we toss it back and forth. He finally catches it then plays keep away with us. Though he is the oldest dog in the group that includes all our children's dogs, he could outrun them all to catch a ball. Recently, we noticed he seemed to have some problems in his hips. Aussies are prone to hip problems because they run so much. We have had to monitor his play because he will continue to run even though he seems to be in pain. He still wants to play catch.

In the winter of 2018 I was loading Doc in my car, he slipped on the ice and twisted his body. He was able to straighten up, but was walking funny. When I got him home I watched him. At first he seemed to be ok, but soon he was walking funny again. We took him to our vet and she said the slip on the ice has caused some pressure on his spine. It's like he threw his back out. He couldn't feel his feet. The vet gave him muscle relaxers and said we may have to look into orthopedic surgery for him.

I had heard there is such a thing as chiropractor vets for animals. I did a little research and found that Sycamore Animal Hospital in the neighboring county does that kind of work. Dr. Sandy Snell was able to see him the day I called.

Doc was kind of nervous in a new place. He kept trying to hide behind me. Sandy sat on the floor with him and sort of cornered him into my legs. It looked like she was petting him, but she was working her hands up his spine. She also appeared to adjust his neck and hips, I think. Aussies have a lot of fur and I just know her hands were somewhere in there. After his first treatment he seemed better. Dr. Snell gave us some supplements and oils to help his joints.

Dr. Snell wanted to see him again in a week. This visit after his massage she used acupuncture on him. He tolerated all of this. We even played fetch and Doc keep away with him while he had the needles in place. Doc Keep Away is where we toss a ball back and forth and he tries to get it. When he does, he plays keep away with us. He brings the ball close but grabs it if you reach for it.

After a couple of months of treatments, we see a big improvement in him. He sometimes still stumbles, and though he can get on furniture but he has adapted how he jumps up. He kind of goes from a seated position instead of jumping from all fours. Sometimes he can get to a place that was difficult for him, like on our bed. We were brushing one of the cats who does not like to be brushed and she was making a lot of noise. Doc loves to chase our cats and always comes running if he hears one yelling. He had not been on our bed since his accident, but let the cat scream and POP! There he is.

Doc continues to be a patient, getting an adjustment every now and then. He is eleven years old and has good quality of life, playing in our backyard and chasing balls and cats.

Alpha

Alpha is the senior cat in our family group. He was adopted from the Humane Society in 2005. Alpha has lived with us through a parade of pets coming and going. He is a big boy, not easily ruffled, seldom if ever letting some whipper snapper of a kitten or dog draw him into confrontation. Usually he just walks on past like he just does not have time to fool with some dumb animal wanting trouble. Most of the time, he is on a bed or sunning himself in the screened porch or the outdoor cat environment.

In the summer of 2018 my son brought his three pit bulls over to play in our fenced yard. Alpha usually ignores the visiting pets. The dogs were on the porch getting a drink when Alpha came through the cat door to lounge in the sun. The cat door is in a sliding glass door to the house and is close to a chest freezer. There is enough room for the cats to comfortably navigate out to the porch with room to spare, but not the dogs. The two young pits saw Alpha and barged over to him with all their power. They are not vicious, just playful, but they do not know their own strength. I heard the noise and ran over there. They had corned Alpha behind the freezer, actually moving it out from the wall. Rather than reach in, I pushed a bunch of recyclables on top of them to distract them long enough to give Alpha a chance to escape. He got around them but they turned and continued to corner him on the side of the freezer. He had been declawed which is lucky for the dogs because Alpha was getting a lot of shots in and would have split their faces.

My son and husband heard the commotion and were able to separate all the animals. Alpha got onto a chair and looked very upset. My son picked him up and looked him over for any injuries. He appeared to have not cuts and could walk and stand, but he was acting very upset and kept low. He went back in the house and hid under a bed. We watched him for a day or so. He seemed off, including not eating well, and not coming up on our bed, which he always does. I decided we need to contact Doc's friend, Sandy at Sycamore.

Sandy looked him over and started to massage him and adjust him. Alpha is a very laid back cat and responded to being handled. He just lay down and enjoyed the attention. After his session, it took a day or so, he was back to his old self. He moves around the house in a kind of easy lope. Even if headed to his food dish, he walks. When he crosses a room, he just moseys along, past our other pets barely giving them a notice. He's just that cool. He appeared to not need a second session, he seemed fine. He was roughed up some by those ding head pits. I said he was run over by a herd of buffalo. But his treatment at Sycamore seemed to set him right.

Fiero

The next pet that I sought help from Sycamore was Fiero, my long haired calico. If Alpha is the King of Cool in our house, Fiero is the Prissy Princess. A few years ago my daughter worked as a kennel assistant at a veterinarian's office near where she attended college. There was a car dealership adjacent to the Vet's office where people regularly dumped animals. They knew the office will take them him, care for them and try to re-home. That's how we got this cat.

She is called Fiero because that is where she was found, in a Fiero. I'm not sure what made my daughter think this, but she felt this little calico needed me. I didn't need her, since I already had a bunch of cats, mostly rescues or drop offs from my children, but somehow she needed me. She is a lovey little cat to me only. I believe in her perfect world, the rest of the world, including my other pets and husband, would vanish and she could just sit in my lap all day.

The dogs easily spook her because she is very vocal. If she wouldn't meow loudly when she comes around, the 2 dogs wouldn't alert and chase her. She also does not like the other cats. If she i on my lap or is thinking about jumping up there, if another car is around, it is a potential cat fight. She will hiss at a cat walking past. One of my cats will challenge her, I believe, for sport. She's very pretty and small and pettable but she only wants me to pet her.

I noticed after having her for awhile that she was not keeping up cleaning her coat. She hadnot always had this problem, so we thought something was wrong. My son and I tried to trim out some mats in her long coat. Of course, she did not cooperate and it was quite a struggle. We saw that he cut her. so we stopped trimming. I was worried about the cut so I called Sandy at Sycamore. Sandy had me bring her in and she found that there was more than on cut from us armatures trimming the mats.

Sandy cleaned up the badly trimmed fur and the cuts we accidentally inflicted on poor little Fiero. She also adjusted her so she can clean her own fur. Fiero really needs an attitude adjustment. She really doesn't like anyone but me and is very vocal about it. At Sycamore there is a cat, named Frank, who seems to be an empath and have some healing powers. He will jump up in your lap or sit next to a pet to comfort while at the office. Of course, that is with everyone except Fiero. Frank assessed Fiero, correctly, I might add, as a brat who does not deserve his care, so he just ignores her. No more than what she deserves, she is a brat. If she can't be nice, then she doesn't need his help. Good for you Frank.

Dodger

We have a tabby cat named Dodger who sneezes all the time. I talked to Sandy about her and she said she might be able to help her. Dodger is also a cool character who rules the roost. She suffers no fools, and if some dog thinks he can chase her, that dog has another think coming. A few dogs have run away with a nasty scratch on his nose and a hard lesson learned. Don't mess with Dodger.

So, Dodger had to be to be coaxed out of her cat carrier with nice words and massages. Unfortunately, Dodger next got to have her sinuses flushed. She was not a big fan of the procedure and resisted some. There was a bit of Dodger fur flying all over the room. Then she got to sit in front of a diffuser with smelly stuff in it and laugh at her arch enemy, Fiero while she gets her treatment. Fiero is a very vocal cat, (remember Prissy Princess?) and made lots of noise and used very unladylike language.

I mentioned Sandy's cat, Frank. He really seems to have some empathy and healing powers. He will come around and sit in your lap if he perceives anxiety, apparently. Well, one morning we miraculously arrived early and were waiting in the car. Doc was getting worked up and nervous in the car. Frank jumped up on the hood of my car and stared at the scared dog. Doc saw his stare and stared back. It really seemed to calm him down. Hopefully, Sandy doesn't start charging for Frank's services.

Leslie Motter

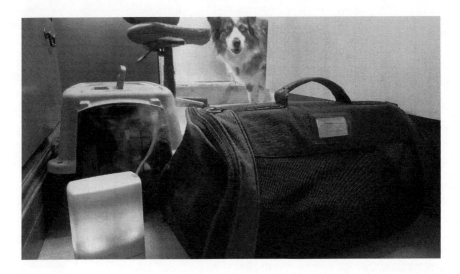

JIM'S STORY

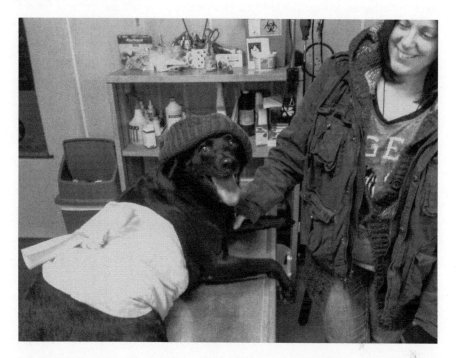

This is the story about my dog Jim and his remarkable recovery thanks to the effort and special care given to him by our one of a kind vet, Sandra Snell.

Jim came to us as a rescue. He is half lab and half jack russell terrier. He was all legs and a little body. When we first got him he was always running, and playing as most puppies do. Then after a few years he started to fill out, well, he got a little overweight. I never really worried about it because he always had so much energy. I just figured he would burn it off.

Jim always liked to sleep in our bed because he was a cuddlebug. He would jump on and off the bed. Morning and night. I never thought he would ever have a problem with it.

One Sunday morning I woke up like normal never thinking this was gonna be a really bad day. Jim was in his usual spot looking at me. I found that unusual because he likes to wake me up with a paw on the face, or kicking my face. He tried to climb up for good morning kisses but I could tell he couldn't. I knew then something was wrong.he couldn't move his lower half. I thought maybe he slept on it wrong and his legs might be asleep. So, I picked him up and set him on the floor. Almost immediately he fell over. I thought "Holy Cow, I broke him." He tried to pull himself across the floor, but all he could manage was dragging his rear end. It was truly a very sad sight. I felt so sorry for him. So I called the only person I knew could help him, I called Sandy. When I told her what was going on she told me to bring him in.

We arrived at her office, I carried his poor broken body into the exam room and laid him on the table. He had even loss control of his bladder. Sandy examined him and came up with the diagnosis. Jim had somehow ruptured a disc in his spine. I believed it was caused from him being overweight and jumping on and off the bed.

She explained that we had three options.

Number 1- I could have him put down. That to me was not even an option. I love my puppy too much to even think of that.

Number 2- he could have sugary done. Which she said is expensive, is very painful for the dog, and sometimes, doesn't always work.

And I asked what was number 3? Because I didn't like the first two. Sandy said if we would let her, she would like to try doing energy work (Reiki), some acupuncture, some stim treatments, and a healing laser. We decided to go with option 3.

So, there began Jim's journey with Sandy. Every day Jim was there for his appointment. Every day she worked on him. Every day it was laser, needles, energy work, repeat. Every day he was carried in and out of the office.

Now, after about a solid month or so of this treatment, we noticed Jim starting to move his back legs a little. We still had to carry him everywhere, in and out to go potty, to his food and water dishes, etc. He never whimpered, or whined, never cried a bit. He was a trooper. Then it was about the end of month 2, beginning of month 3, we were sitting in the living room, I will never forget this as long as I live, Jim just stood up off of his bed in the living room, looked at me, and WALKED into the kitchen! I could not believe my eyes! This poor, broken creature whom we had been carrying around for almost 3 months, just got up and WALKED across the floor! I almost started crying. I just kept saying to myself, "it's working, it's working, he's gonna be ok!"

Jim continued his treatments everyday for a while after that. Then it went to once or twice a week, then to a few times a month. That was a few years ago. Jim still sees Sandy, but it's on an as needed basis.

Everytime I see him outside now, running and playing and rough housing with our other dogs or the grandkids, I can't help but send up a small, silent prayer for the gift that God gave to the world in giving Sandy the healing gifts that she has. Jim is not 100 percent yet, when he runs it's not exactly in a straight line, it's a little sideways, but I don't care, he can run and play, and that's what puppies are supposed to do.

I know there are a lot of people out there who would not have taken option number 3. They're to busy or don't have the patience it takes to care for an injured pound puppy that is broken. Many people would of chosen option number 1 and I feel very sad for those people.

If you bring an animal into your life, especially a shelter animal, it is YOUR responsibility to provide that animal with a good, quality life. These animals are NOT expendable.

Jim has brought so much love into our home, and has been there for me through some of the most difficult times in my life. He doesn't care if I cry on him, his fur has soaked up many of my tears. He just looks at me with his ears perked up, and through his big, brown eyes as if to say "I'm here for you dad, you were there for me, now I'm here for you, I got you." That is more than I could have ever asked for.

Many thank yous go out to Sandy........for giving me my Jim back.

May God bless you and keep you safe.

Sincerely,
SHAWN MARSCHKE.

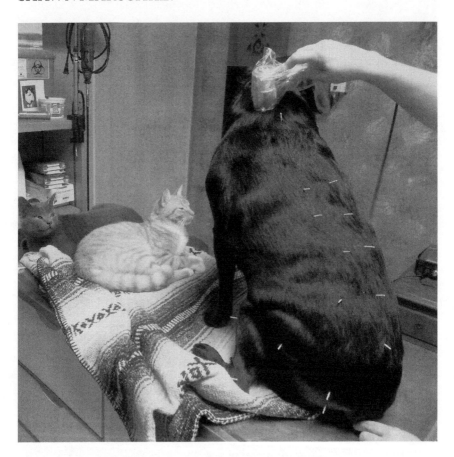

WILLIAMS' FAMILY STORY

This is our youngest Lab, Kong. He was born with severe Hip Dysplasia and joint problems. We were told by a veterinarian he would have to be euthanized or have both hips replaced at over $5000/hip and that he could still have problems. We were heartbroken. We didn't want to lose him or have him live in the kind of pain we were told he would have, but we didn't have that kind of money.

My brother told us about a veterinarian in Sycamore, Ohio that is a chiropractor for animals. That Veterinarian is Dr. Sandra Snell at Sycamore Animal Hospital. We called her and explained our situation and she made us an appointment. We were asked to bring our fur baby's X Rays with us. Dr. Snell had us look at the X Rays with her and showed us all his problems. She said he might not live a full life span but she could help and he wouldn't have to be euthanized. Now, thanks to the therapy, chiropractic adjustments and the medication she gives him, our baby boy is going to be 8 yrs. old July 21, 2018 and is doing great ! He's spoiled rotten and runs and jumps like a normal dog. <3

Dr. Snell also cares for our other two Labs, 9 and 10 yrs. old, they have age related back and hip problems. We were surprised when we took our 9 yr. old to her. He never liked going to the vet. He would get to the door going in and stop and sit down and we couldn't get him to move. My husband would lift him up and in through the doorway and he still wouldn't move. He had to coax and practically drag him into the office. At Dr. Snell's office he walks right in the door and right into the office without any hesitation and acts like he's at home. She sits on the floor with them while gently giving them so much care, love and attention. They all love her and love going there. <3

Dr. Snell not only offers Holistic Healing for pets but people as well. During a visit to her office for a treatment for our youngest Lab, Dr. Snell asks us, "Which one of you is having neck pain?" My husband and I looked at each other, not sure how she knew but she did. I answered that I have had neck and shoulder pain for over 20 years. I had been seeing doctors and a chiropractor through the years with very little relief. She looked up at me and said, "I can help you with that." I have to say after having pain for so many years I was doubtful, but at this point I was willing to try almost anything. I had times when I had been so dizzy I had to get on the floor and crawl somewhere to lay down until the dizziness passed. I agreed to let her try. She took me into a dimly lit room and had me lie down on a padded table. The lighting, the smell, the entire atmosphere of that room relaxed me so much I wanted to go to sleep. She did massage therapy on my neck and shoulder and with some adjustment within 30 minutes or so I felt better than I had felt in over 20 years ! It was instant relief !! Now, I can look up at the sky and not worry about getting dizzy or falling down, I can move my head in all directions without pain. Dr. Sandra Snell is an amazing person and doctor. She has improved the quality of life for all of us. My husband and I can't thank her enough for the loving care she has given our family. <3

Forever Thankful,
Dean and Beckie Williams

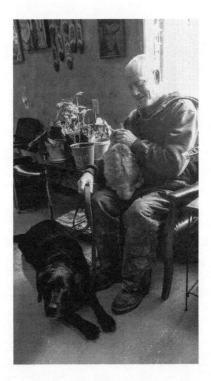

SHAMROCK, TAM, AND CHRISTINA'S STORY

Sandy changed my life, and while that might sound like a cliché and sweeping generic accolade, it is the only way to express what her presence in my life has meant to me.

I first met Sandy in 2009, when my 3 ½ year old cat, Shamrock was dying. She had a congenital heart defect, and her life was coming to an end, but I wanted to know if there was anything else that could be done for her. On the recommendation of a colleague, I drove to Sycamore, Ohio and met Sandy for the first time. On a strange whim, I had brought Shamrock's sister, Tam, along. (I think I was afraid that if Shamrock's condition was congenital, then her littermate might have it as well.)

There was little to be done for Shamrock, and we knew that her days were few, but Sandy assured me that she was in no pain, so we were prepared to take her home. When she examined Tam, my husband and I were sitting in the waiting room, but were in earshot. After a long period of silence, Sandy said, "Tam's been hurt."

I was shocked. I had no idea that Tam was in pain. Stunned, I asked from the other room, "How did she get hurt?"

Another long pause. "She doesn't want to say."

My husband and I looked at each other. Was this for real? "Tam-Tam, tell the nice doctor what's going on," I said.

Long pause. "She doesn't want to get anyone in trouble."

More astonishment from us both. "Tam-Tam, no one's going to get in trouble. You need to tell the doctor right now how you got hurt."

Very long pause. Sandy said, "Who's Brian?"

All the hair stood up on my body, as we gaped at each other. We had never met this woman, never told her anything except about the health and history of the cats. Brian was a college student who was living with us at the time. We were having some issues with his attitude and were ready for him to leave. Sandy told us that Brian had kicked Tam, injuring her hind-quarters. I knew at that moment that Sandy had a unique ability to communicate and heal, and I wanted to learn as much as I could from her.

I had recently taken a Level I Reiki class, but I did not feel a strong connection with my instructor. I wanted to continue my Reiki studies, and Sandy agreed to help me make that happen. I spent time with her, observing and assisting her with her animal and human clients. We did this work both in her clinic in Sycamore and on the road, where we mostly worked on horses and their humans. She taught me to trust in my intuition, something that had been a struggle for my over-intellectualizing brain. She helped me understand the importance of learning the rules and also to know when to break them. Her approach was free from much of the dogma and constraint that I had found in my previous Reiki training, and my skills as a Reiki practitioner grew quickly. I opened my own practice, and when I became a Reiki Master, I started teaching students myself, with a deep grounding in gratitude for the lessons and experience I had gained with Sandy. The gift of her knowledge and time is truly one of the most precious gifts I have ever received, and it was given with great love and generosity of spirit, which is her essence. Reiki has transformed my life in all the best ways possible, and I credit much of that to my teacher and soul-sister, Sandy Snell.

Christina Laberge, DMA, Reiki Master Teacher
www.wellspringenergyworks.com

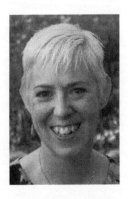

LYON'S FAMILY STORY

By Megan Lyons

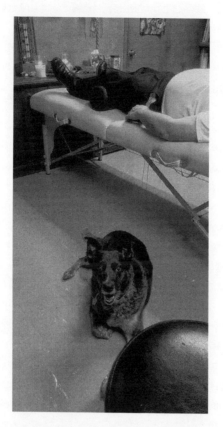

My story with Dr. Snell began with my family and our dog. When our dog, Maggie, stopped using her back legs suddenly we did what everyone does. We tried all the traditional veterinary medicine, and nothing seemed to work. Eventually, we were pointed towards Dr. Snell. Once Maggie started alternative medicine therapy, within a month we went from having to carry our dog around with a towel supporting her hind legs to her walking around like nothing ever happened. This lead to my father going to Dr. Snell as a healer whenever he was feeling out of sorts. You can tell the difference in him after an appointment, as he stands straighter, his movements are smoother, and he has better circulation. Seeing the difference in my father and my dog, I became curious about alternative medicine, and that is what led me into my ongoing journey with Dr. Snell. After shadowing her for some time, I decided to go through with my first attunement. After that I was more sensitive to things around me, and because of shadowing with Dr. Snell I understood more about how energy healing worked.

I was diagnosed this past year with a blood clot in a sinus of my brain that was completely blocking blood flow out of one side of my head. While I was in the hospital, I remember vividly when I felt Dr. Snell working on me. I was laying there in the dark, no TV, no sounds, because any light or noise was excruciating at that point. I was debating if I could fall asleep without asking for any more pain medication because I was scared that I would get addicted to it. Then I started heating up, like someone had wrapped me in a blanket they just pulled from the dryer. Only the warmth was building from the inside out, and I sighed in relief because with the warmth also came an ease in the pain. My mother told me that my father had mentioned to Dr. Snell what had happened to me, and I told my mother that I felt her working on me. The next day, after five days of not leaving a bed, I got up and took a shower. So, from miles and miles away, Dr. Snell gave me the healing I needed. It doesn't stop there though, for months after that I was on a balancing act of medications, pain, and more medications. Eventually, I was tired of being in pain, and having the concentration span of a squirrel while trying to go to class. So, I forced time into my schedule and went to Dr. Snell. Within two Reiki treatments, I was back to feeling normal again and was able to stop the medications.

This year, my ninety-year old grandfather was taken to the hospital suddenly for dehydration and weakness. When my mother left to take him to the hospital, she left without telling me. Shortly after her leaving, I woke up and felt the strong urge to burn sage and light a candle. While doing this, my father came into my room and told me what was happening. I focused on my grandfather's healing, and instead of worrying, I concentrated on the love I had for him. My mother said that the doctors found an obstruction, but within twenty-four hours it had resolved itself without surgery. This technique is something that I learned from Dr. Snell.

BART'S STORY

By Mary Jo Bish and has been printed in many Dog Magazines to Help Educate, Give Hope, and even Save Lives.

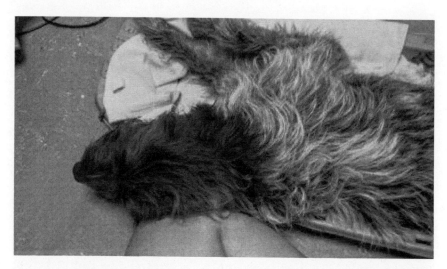

August 2, 2015 Jerry and I left to visit his mother. The dogs had been fed and exercised as usual and were in their runs or crates. Our daughter, Rebecca, checked on everyone at noon and all was well. We came home around 6PM and found Bart paralyzed in his crate. He could blink and wag his tail, his head bobbled around out of control. Other than that, he could move nothing. Bart was confused but in no pain. We called a family friend, Javier, to help get Bart out of the crate. On the other phone, we contacted our veterinarian who has done emergencies in the past. He was unavailable but the answering machine told us an emergency clinic was covering for him. Javier and Jerry put Bart on a toboggan sled and carried him out to the car. I rode in the back to comfort Bart and make sure he didn't get rolled out of the sled. Our 40 minute drive took less than 30 and because we called ahead, the techs were waiting for us. Before we were allowed to take Bart inside, we were asked for the $90 fee for exam. That shocked us. Inside, the young vet said, "Your dog is paralyzed." The thought "No joke, Jack." went through my head. He began to examine Bart's ears. I asked for an x-ray of the neck and back. He responded that he needed to give the dog a physical first. Protocol he said. Bart was no longer moving his head at all and we knew he was losing his battle. I demanded an x-ray. The vet agreed at this time and rolled Bart, sled and all, away. The vet returned with the x-ray and without Bart, and began showing us the intestines, stomach and so on. When asked where Bart was, he replied that since Bart was paralyzed, he had left him in the back. Internally I was furious but I just firmly asked the vet to go get Bart. He did. Upon return he again began to show us internal organs. We stopped him, reminded him our 40+ years involvement in dogs, and asked him to concentrate on the spinal area. There were no compressed discs, no signs of arthritis, nothing out of the ordinary. The vet said he needed to make a consultation phone call. Fifteen minutes later he returned and informed us that Bart needed to stay at the clinic overnight for observation, then we could pick him up and take him to Ann Arbor to a neurological specialist for another consultation. This vet had no idea what was wrong with Bart. We were informed at this point that the overnight stay would be $850 payable up front and the consultation tomorrow would be $300. If the neurological vet felt surgery was necessary, it would be $3000-$4000 with no guarantee. I asked what this clinic would be doing for Bart if we left him there. The response was priceless, "We would observe him." We took Bart home. Once home, Bart's eyes sparkled a bit more. He seemed to understand that we would be doing everything we could for him. We piled soft beds on the floor for him. I rested on the floor next to him. Whenever I knew Bart was awake, I massaged his legs and helped him do "bicycles". I had no idea what I was doing and whether or not I was making things worse but doing something seemed to make Bart more alert. I put water on his tongue but he had a tough time trying to make a swallowing motion. Lots of tears and prayers on my part. My vet was still unavailable on that Monday. So we called our holistic vet, Dr. Sandy Snell, in Sycamore, Ohio and told her what was going on. She cleared as much of her schedule as she could and told us to come right away. She met us at the door and helped us carry the sled and Bart inside. We had consulted Dr. Snell once before with a pregnant Griff who was absolutely refusing to eat anything. With an adjustment and some oils, Bella began eating right away. We hoped Dr. Snell would know what to do in this case.

Dr. Snell sat on the floor to examine Bart briefly. She then proceeded to place acupuncture needles on opposite sides of Bart's spine from tail to occiput. After a short rest she ran a cold laser beside and between the needles. Bart could again move his head albeit not in a controlled manner. When the needles were removed, she applied essential oils and did deep massage. Following the massage was a chiropractic adjustment near the hip area and mid spine. By the time we left, Bart could move his legs somewhat and his tail was moving again. He was able to keep himself upright on his chest (sternal) for a few moments before returning to his side. Dr. Snell did not immediately have a diagnosis, but at least we saw improvement with what she did during the 4 hours she worked on him. When we returned home, Bart and sled were carried to rest in the shade of a large maple tree. He ate pieces of cheese! We set up the whelping pen which is 4x8 in the breezeway for Bart. This was easy for us to get in and out of and gave Bart lots of room to scoot around in. By the third day, Bart crawled through the grass about 3 feet to get to Jerry. He was really tired after that. He did eat half of his regular food that day. August 6th (Day 5) Bart returned to Dr. Snell's for a repeat treatment. He seemed less confused when we left. She sent home essential oils for us to use every morning and night and showed us how to massage him. We needed to restrain him in the sled by this time because he kept trying to get up when we were moving him. August 8 (Day 7) Bart staggered to his feet and attempted to wander around in the two x-pens we had set up under the tree. He fell often but kept trying. Dr. Snell said he had great courage! August 9 (Day 8) Bart walked in his drunken manner from the x-pen to the sidewalk that leads around our house. We called out to him to slow down but he kept going. We had to trot to catch him. We don't think he could reverse himself once he got moving. Bart now always had to be restrained in the sled when getting him in the car. That did not make him happy! We did not want to lift him for fear of damaging whatever was causing this problem. Bart visited Dr. Snell three and sometimes four times a week for acupuncture and laser treatments. These were always followed by massage and sometimes adjustments. We felt Bart was getting stiff from living in the whelping box. So he got his freedom and the breezeway became his. His massages became a twice a day routine. We'd laugh because when Bart saw the container with the oils in it, he'd wobble over to the couch to get his treatment. His tongue would dart in and out of his mouth as the oils were massaged into his body. We knew he was enjoying this part of the treatment. Bart got a special play yard within the fenced area for our other Griffs. Thus, he could be with them without getting jumped on. Spoiled or loved? Near the end of August, we got a phone call from a former puppy purchaser, Brett Kinkaid DVM. He lives in Oklahoma and had called to tell us news about the pup he had purchased. So I told him about Bart since his puppy was Bart's grandson. He told us he thought we had a case of FCE (fibrocartilagenous embolism). His diagnosis was based on the fact that Bart had not evidenced any pain. Of course, we had not heard of FCE and began our research. FCE is a stroke-like event within the spinal cord: symptoms are very sudden in onset and vary with the location of the FCE. Small particles of fibrocartilage believed to come from the discs between the vertebrae block blood vessels within the spinal cord. It is not related to disc herniations. FCE typically results from an injury to the spinal cord often caused when a dog jumps or lands awkwardly. The type of dog most likely to be affected by FCE is a young or middle-aged athletic dog of medium size. Pain is usually present initially but not present after onset. As far as we know, Bart experienced no pain at any time. Symptoms can include sudden severe pain that makes the dog cry or yelp followed by lessening pain after a few minutes, signs of weakness; partial to full paralysis of a rear limb; a wobbly or uncoordinated gait; and lack of pain response after initial signs of painfulness, yet the dog still can't use his body normally. Bart could not move himself at all. The treatment for FCE even with animals with a poor prognosis due to swelling or decreased pain sensation is to begin immediate and aggressive physical therapy. Studies show that physiotherapy beginning immediately after diagnosis can have a major influence on recovery. This should include hydrotherapy, as well as acupuncture, laser therapy, neuromuscular electrical stimulation, range of motion exercises, massage and supplements (B vitamins, NAC N-acetylcysteine, vitamin E and ALA alpha-lipoic acid). Aggressive treatment of this acute condition can be very rewarding. Implementing an immediate rehabilitation program is your dog's best option for a full recovery. Left untreated 80% of the dogs do not recover enough to have a second chance at life. By early spring Bart's visits to Dr. Snell were needing to be fewer and fewer. He does miss the car rides and the hamburger on the way home, I'm sure. Although Bart continues to improve, his butt still bounces off the walls in the hallway when he is too excited to control everything. He surprised us once by rising from a sitting position without support to put his front feet on the shoulders of a friend! It has only been 11 months since his trial began. He has come a long way in that time.

Bart finished his championship very easily. At six months in his first two shows he won majors by going over specials. He loved to show and is the sire of four champions. We promised Bart and ourselves that if he continued to improve, we would enter him in another dog show. We would tell his story to others in hopes of educating them about FCE. What better place than at the first AWPGA supported entry at Ann Arbor Kennel Club on July 9, 2016?

Jerry and Mary Jo Bish and Bart

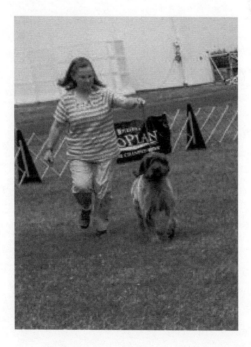

Medical information was taken from: Healthy Pets with Dr. Karen Becker
http://healthypets.mercola.com/sites/healthypets/archive/2013/06/03/
fibrocartilaginous-embolism.aspx
Affiliated Veterinary Specialists http://www.avsspecialists.com/client-
resources/articles/ fibrocartilaginous-embolism-fce/

BELLA'S STORY

By Nancy Wilson 5/15/18

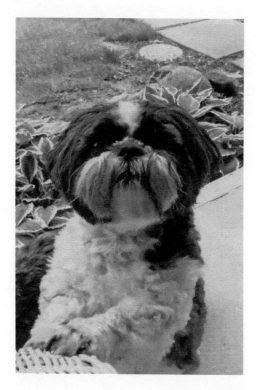

Bella's story really begins before her birth - a little background to illustrate how much this dog means to me: Back in 2008 I was happily living with three dogs, a Yorkshire terrier, Jasper who was 10, a Norfolk terrier, Toby, also 10 and a Shih Tzu, Mojo, who was 4. He was my "hope for the future", as I knew that my terriers were getting older. What happened to me at that time completely devastated me. You see, I lost two of my three beloved furry children in less than a week; Toby died of heart failure, and, five days later Mojo, my four year old shih tzu died of autoimmune hemolytic anemia. I was completely devastated. After several months of crying endlessly, both at home and at work, I sought help from my doctor. I just couldn't stop grieving. For the only time in my life, I relied on the antidepressants she prescribed. I took them for two years, and then stopped, which was the hardest part. I will never take them again. Mojo was purchased from a "backyard breeder", so, thinking to research a better breeder this time around, I spent a year looking and researching to find a good breeder.

I found a breeder in Pennsylvania whose line included many many champions; some of which were at Westminster. We made the trip to pick out our pup - pet quality, since we don't get involved in showing. All we wanted was to love and cherish a healthy shih tzu. We brought our beautiful girl, Bella, home and delighted in her.

All was going well, until the spring of 2011, when Bella, now two years old began straining when having a bowel movement. Blood started showing up in her feces, and I immediately took her to our local veterinarian, who did an exam, including x-rays. When they couldn't find anything, they referred me to The Akron Veterinary Hospital where there are specialists available for almost any condition. They quickly determined Bella had a rectal tumor which they surgically removed and sent off to determine if it was benign or malignant. The doctor told me that I shouldn't worry, as many times, these things are benign and he was pretty sure that would be the case. It wasn't long before I got the call that no one wants to get, with the worst news possible.

Bella's tumor was malignant, and the prognosis was terrible. I was told that she would only live another three months - and that only if we went ahead with chemo and radiation treatment. To say I was devastated, yet again, is the understatement of all time. I was heartsick. Each day I felt like I was waking up to a nightmare. Besides the cost of chemo and radiation, I was only too aware of what quality of life would be like for her.

That point was the beginning of our miracle. I phoned a very good groomer who I remembered had told me the name of a holistic veterinarian, Dr. Sandy Snell, in Sycamore, Ohio. I phoned and made an appointment to take Bella to see her as soon as possible. I took all of Bella's medical paperwork from the Akron clinic, including the surgery to remove the tumor and the dire prognosis. Dr. Snell sat down with us and took the time to read through all the paperwork thoroughly, and then said the words that dared let me hope again, for the first time since the nightmare began: "I can't promise that it will help, but I CAN promise it will do no harm". So began the weekly, then semi-weekly, then monthly trips to Sycamore Animal Hospital. We live an hour and a half away, so we would go every Saturday and the healing began in earnest, with Reiki energy treatments and a whole host of other alternative treatments given by this very gifted, psychic empath, Dr. Snell. Needless to say, Bella loved the treatments, which were completely non invasive and WAY better than chemo and radiation. She would come out of those appointments and we would go for long hikes, stopping at the parks on the way home.

Now the greatest part of the story: Bella improved and improved after each visit and her quality of life just got better and better! At first, and to be honest, for a long time, really, I constantly watched over her, worrying and fretting every time we went out to the yard to go potty. I watched for any straining, or bloody stools, absolutely terrified the tumor would come back, and so, too, the nightmare of losing her. Now, the most amazing part of Bella's story: She is nine years old!!!!! She has never had any ill health at all since seeing Dr. Snell, and I call her a walking, living, breathing miracle. This beautiful little girl was given only three months to live, with a treatment plan that would have assured her no good quality of life, and now she is nine years old and loves to hike and toss her pretty head like she's a pup!

I have often wondered if we had gone ahead with the chemo and radiation treatments, would we have been able to go for long hikes after these appointments? I think not. Indeed, she would not be with us today. I have learned a lot from this whole experience: western medicine may be great for patching people and animals up and setting broken bones, but it certainly can, and does, fall far short when it comes to absolute healing. Dr. Snell can communicate with animals in a way no one else I've ever met can. Since this happened, I have done a lot of research on psychic healing, energy work, long distance healing, etc. I have found that you don't even have to believe in it, and it STILL works. I thank God (spirit), every day that I made the call for help to this amazing, gifted healer who literally saved the life of my beautiful little miracle girl, Bella.

ZOE'S STORY

By Colleen Vallo 5/29/18

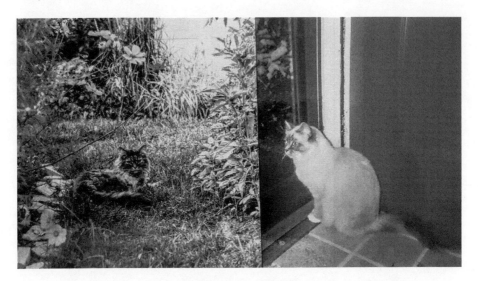

Kitty Cat on left. Zoe or Kitty Cat Come Back on right.

I lost my dear little Zoe, but it was in the best way possible—through Dr. Sandra Snell's loving assistance. When I took Zoe to Dr. Snell that early Monday morning, it was to get fluids and then take her back home. But Zoe had other plans. She told Dr. Snell, who is an animal communicator, that she was sick and tired of being sick and tired. My eyes opened to her real condition, and I knew I couldn't fight it. It was time to leave her little four-pound body that had fought hard through kidney disease ravages.

Dr. Snell first worked on Zoe using reiki to clear her and assist her transition. I believe in animals' ability to reincarnate, and Dr. Snell worked on her to remove karma and the energetic essences of her kidney disease. When she reincarnated as Zoe from my former cat, Kitty Cat, she seemed to bring in the very diseases that afflicted Kitty even though Zoe was in a brand new body.

When Dr. Snell finished, Zoe and I went to a room where she does attunements for reiki clearings on humans. I held Zoe as she worked on me. I never felt such peace, even though I was torn up with grief. Afterward, I remained in the reiki room while Dr. Snell euthanized Zoe. I couldn't participate in that part. I was never rushed. It wasn't the quick in, administer the shot and back out the door that I experienced when I euthanized Kitty Cat. She even gave Zoe and me some homeopathic ignatia to take the "dagger out" of the heart, which it did.

Though Zoe had to go, her passing could not have been more kind and comforting. Dr. Snell did that. While euthanizing our beloved fur babies is never easy, it can be less traumatic and freeing on the body, mind, spirit for everyone. I highly recommend Dr. Snell's veterinary care that includes reiki attunements for animals and her shamanic reiki attunements for people.

Acknowledgement

I am a LIGHT being, I am currently going through a human existence. I can't heal everything. I can't teach everyone. I can't fix everything. But this does not stop me from trying. I will continue to provide the frequency to do this to the best of my ability. What others choose to do with this is up to them.

Greatest Gratitude and Blessings to all of the 4 legged, 2 legged and no legged seen and unseen that has knowingly and unknowingly helped me in this LABOR of LOVE creating this book into reality.

For all things on my path, including myself, past, present, and future in all realms, dimensions, and realities please Forgive Me. I am Sorry. I Respect you. You are Enough. Thank you. God Bless You. You are LOVED BY ME.

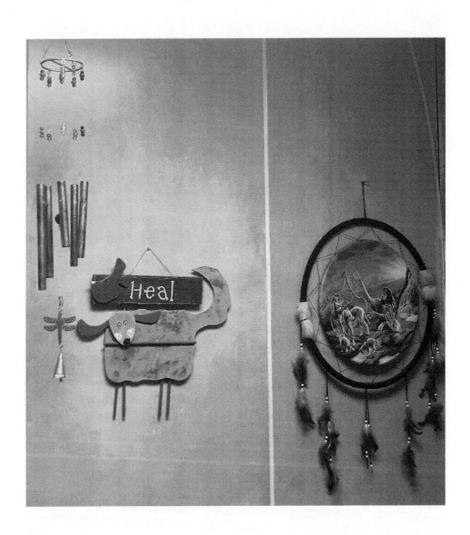

Foreword

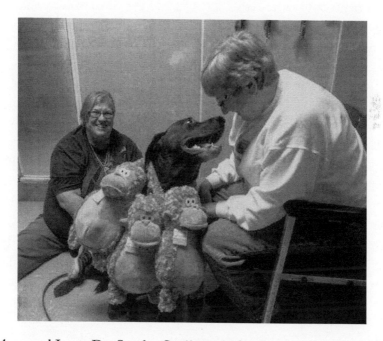

Melton and I met Dr. Sandra Snell just before his surgery for an ACL tear on his right hind leg. Following his surgery, she came with her laser to help him to heal quicker. Shortly after his surgery, he injured his back while he was attempting to chase a cat. As Sandy treated Melton using Reiki, laser, chiropractic, acupuncture, as well as remote distance healing; Melton became stronger and many of his back issues disappeared. Throughout his treatments, Sandy and I began to explore options for me such as attunements, Reiki training, aromatherapy, and so much more.

Each time that I had an adjustment, attunement, and a treatment; Melton was part of the procedure. It was not long until it was apparent that he, too, was becoming a Reiki trained and quite a healer in his own rite. As we all learned to travel together, Melton became more and more attuned to the needs of those we were going to visit. He truly enjoyed being part of the team.

Dr. Sandy became our friend, our mentor, our guide, and our very present healer. Melton would even call her on the phone to request adjustments and attention. She was always available to share her knowledge and her wisdom with us. The various topics that she has written about in this book, she has honed in her own practice and has included us in the process.

Even through I was the least of the healers when I was a part of this threesome, I was privileged to be a member of the team. Sandy and Melton shared their thoughts and ideas equally with me as well as often asked for my input. Each time Dr. Sandy encountered a new theory or technique, she would test it thoroughly with her spirit guides before she would use it in any of her healings. She would also patiently explain the processes and procedures to all who were willing to hear. Each layer of knowledge and wisdom fit so well together to provide for more effective and efficient healing of body, mind, soul, and spirit. All of the techniques and practices that are in this book are truly successful in different areas of the healing realm.

One of the most important things that I have learned from Dr. Sandy is that even though one technique works perfectly for her, it must be fine-tuned for each individual healer before it can be effectively used. The healing comes in so many forms but in all situations, Sandy's methods are just a starting point for a healer. These techniques must be internalized and become an intimate part of the individual putting them into practice.

Each of you will be most pleased that you picked up this book and allowed it to become a part of your being. Internalize its message and practice the material shared within these pages. With your spirit guides, your faith, your confidence, and your willingness to go outside of the everyday norms; you will be able to accomplish so much more than what you ever dreamed possible. Of course, that is how this Universe expects all things to happen. Happy reading and happy healing!

Sharon Neifer, Melton, Chip Paul, and the Cats

Preface

I am often asked, how long have you been doing this type of healing? My most favorite and truthful answer is, "This is not my first life time doing it!!!"

I have always felt pushed to heal every person and every animal entirely and all at once. I have made many lists or forms along the way to try to accomplish this. Most of which shall be included in order of which they are written so you may find what works for you and yours. These things could be used on man or beast because we are all energetic beings. All of these could be done in private without the loved one knowing or in direct contact in public. Whenever given the choice of hands-on or distant healing, I would pick hands on. However, distant healing can be just as powerful, sometimes possible more and always safer. This is why my first book will be about Distant Healing.

I am blessed with a beloved child. She often does not fit into any box, which I am sure genetics play a large part of. I would love to share some of the lessons I have learned along my path to help others. My goal is to give ideas and many things you could do for yourself and loved ones in need besides fundamental prayer and worrying. Thank you, for following your inner compass on some level to find this with Divine Timing when you need it most.

Please always follow your heart, first and always. I am addicted to learning. I also admit there are worse things to be addicted to.... I am always waiting for that one piece of information that helps makes other things I know make sense. I combine this and that or change it around like pieces of a puzzle. Someone draws a line in the sand, I am one of the first to jump over it or question why can't that be done. Mind over matter and all. If it won't harm and might help, then why not try????? These are words I live by every day. My favorite Chinese proverb is "The person who says it cannot be done, should not interrupt the person doing it."

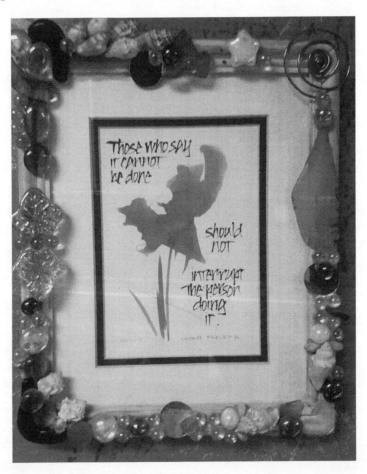

Try doing this exercise if you don't know what your heart wants. First, tell yourself, you love something you love deeply. Sit with that for a moment, how do you feel??? Then try telling yourself, you hate the same exact thing. Can you even do that? Notice how your chest feels, can you breathe? Now you know how your heart can tell you what is right or best for you.

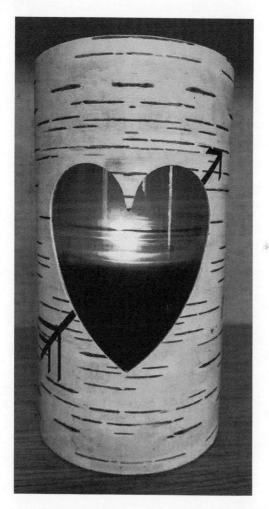

What I will relay here forth is only my version of the truth at this moment in time, space, and reality. Not everything presented to me has agreed with my heart. I do not expect or even pretend, that all of my truths will match all of yours. Many of my old truths no longer match with my new truths as I grow and evolve. I do pray, that as I do my best not to judge others for having different truths then myself, that you may be able to do the same for me. I send you Blessings of Love, Light, and Healing either way.

For the reader consider this my version of Cliff Notes for many of my teachers. There is so much I have learned, if I put everything down there you would not be able to carry this book. I will do my best to be brief but yet still relay the importance of what and why it was to me. References will be listed, so if that piece of a puzzle resonates with you, feel free to springboard off to follow your quest for knowledge and Bliss.

For my teachers thank you for sharing what has been given to you from whatever source. Thank you for reminding me of what I once knew because we are all one, but have forgotten for so many reasons. The hardest lesson for me to teach my students is that all the answers are already within you because just as the Universe mirrors, it is the hardest thing for me to remember myself......

AHO

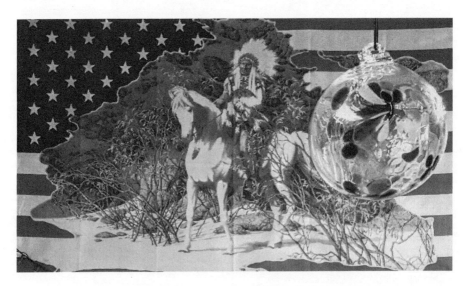

Prayer Warrioring

Prayer Warrior

"From Wikipedia, the free encyclopedia
Prayer warrior is a term used by many evangelical and other Christians to
refer to anyone who is committed to praying for others.

Within the context of Dominion theology, prayer warriors see themselves as
engaged in spiritual warfare against satanic forces.[1]

Prayer warriors may pray for individuals, or for entire states or regions. One
recent development has been prayer undertaken by groups of people flying over
the areas for which they wish to undertake intercession.[2]

References
Stephen Hunt, Christian Millenarianism: from the Early Church to Waco
(Indiana University Press, 2001), p. 60 online.
Sharon Coolidge, "'Prayer Warriors' take to the sky for salvation", Cincinnati.
com, 6 April 2007".

I have been told by many Angels that, "The best way to confront Darkness is to raise the Light. If you go in expecting a battle, a battle is what you will receive. As the vibration rises, the lower vibrations leave."

Prayers are the Love, Light or Action to raise the vibration.

Warrioring is not, in this case, the Battler, but the process of Light Working.

Prayer Warrioring is holding the LOVE & LIGHT and sending it farther and larger than imaged. Atomic Love Bombs.

Awesomeness Cubed wording has been given to me to use longer then I can remember. One night after doing a 3rd Eye Opener YouTube video all night long, Spirit (my Guides, Angels, Inner Voice, Creator, etc.) reminded me I had been given my daughter's name more than 20 years before she was born. And so too was Awesomeness Cubed the name that had come way before the physical thing was here in reality. Later Spirit explained why it is Cubed and it is revealed later in this book.

Spirit told me to write about "Lessons Learned" when I first started putting things together to create this book. I am very Grateful I started with that and not Awesomeness Cubed...

Holistic — Wholistic

To me, this means to treat the Whole problem or Whole being. I went to Veterinary School to help animals in need. Once I was in practice for a while and started down my holistic path, a big Aha moment came and Spirit concurred. Animals often feel they are here to help their people. So many clients come in saying you are not going to believe this, but we both have..... Or I have had many pets die of this same thing... I believe it more than they will ever know.

After I started doing Reiki, I would work on the owners and the animals would get better!!!! So I built a "Human Reiki Room" at the Clinic. I keep learning and adding help for man and beast or the WHOLE FAMILY. Thereby changing the whole world.

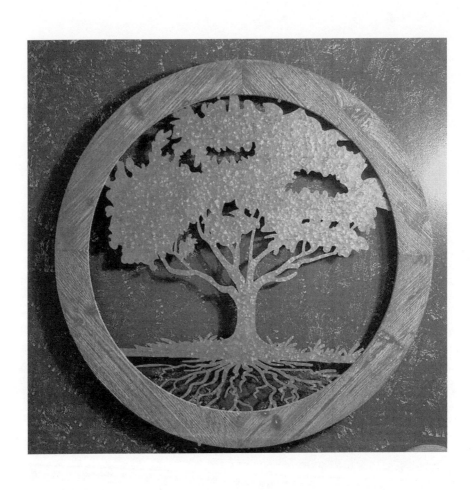

Distant Healing

My mother made me do it.....
After Veterinary School I moved to another state in 1/1994. Mommers, my mom, would tell me there would be something wrong with one of her critters. In the beginning, she would at least tell me which one, but later she would not even give me that intel. My mission, which I always excepted was figuring out all the W's (who, what, where, when, why) and how to fix it. This was way before smartphones, instant messaging, and video chatting. It was also before I knew how to check in with my Guides or did Animal communication. I just had to feel my body, focus on a critter, and then feel where and how my body felt different. And so my empathic skills were born and trained. I would report back to Mommers my findings and recommendations. Often the issue would be resolved.

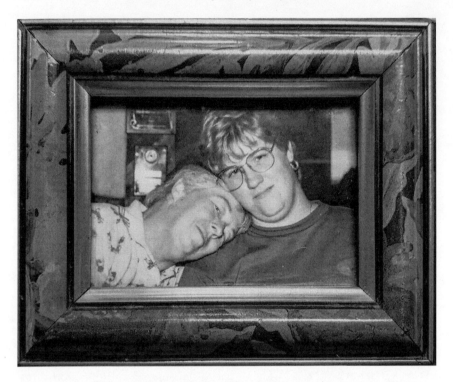

Time and space are merely an illusion. When my daughter was young, she walked in and asked what I was doing?. I told her I was working on a dog on the other side of the Earth in Australia. A Chiropractor owned this dog. The dog had its second anterior cruciate ligament (ACL) injury. The first ACL was treated surgically. The owner wanted to know if the current ACL could be treated holistically or required another surgery. I think I had a picture to help me connect to this dog. I felt the changes in my body. I communicated to this dog, and he said yes to everything I asked. So I threw a trick question in the mix, Are you a cat? Yes. So then I pictured an ACL surgery from a dog's view. Then I asked again, do you want another ACL surgery? A colossal NO came through as his response. I wrote up my findings and sent out an email via dial up to the owner. I went to play with my daughter. A couple of hours later I returned to the computer to see the owner had responded. She asked what had I done because her dog who had not moved for some time, got up, picked up a toy, went outside, ran and played. I replied they were saying NO to surgery!

One more of my distant healing/reading stories. This client was probably 300 miles away. I had gone through all of my testing, recommendations, and healings that I had at that time (I keep learning, adding, and growing). This client took the dog to her regular human chiropractor and then called me. I have to tell the Chiropractor were the problems are and how to adjust the dog. At one point I said the right hip is low. The Chiropractor got upset and said No the left hip is high. I explain to him I am so many miles away, where he has hands on the dog, and that the pelvis is a box so Right hip low is about the same thing as Left hip high...

One of the best things about distant healing is it can be done anonymously. The sender will have the release of Ego and fulfillment of service. The vast majority of people will not be able to trace back who was sending the help, which can take a lot of the pressure for perfection off of the sender. The intended receiver is not thrown into the this can't help mindset or No-sibo effect. Anonymous distant healing is a win-win for the sender and intended receiver. So this might be the best way to get started or bring Random Acts of Kindness to a whole new level.

Many Healing Techniques state, require or highly recommend that permission is given from the intended receiver. The following is my current way to leap over that line in the sand: Permission is asked for this to be done. If denied, by the intended receiver, permission is asked again to their "Higher Selves." If denied again, continue for yourself. The only one you can truly change is yourself. However, since we are all One, by improving yourself, hopefully, the intended receiver will also benefit..... Or by looking at it from Ho'oponopono theory, you take full responsibility for everything and everyone, so working on yourself, will help others....

The sender should send Love for the greatest good of all. Before you work on others with any of my projects, you should use it on yourself first. My projects are extensive. Often the brain may shut down because there is so much to process. I have had many people fall asleep or say they could not hear during a reading. So I have found it helpful just to take the conscious brain out of the process by holding their neck during a Reiki session and silently reading a list. Or possibly just do it distantly. When I channel, I will often speak in tongues. I believe this is, so our conscious mind does not override the work, by saying it is not possible. Be open to the possibility of White Light, unconditional LOVE, and Perfect Health. Which was my first Spirit given Reiki mantra.

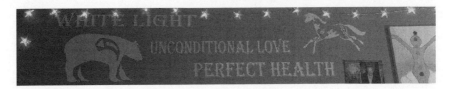

Have faith. Just because you or your intended receiver could not feel the change, does not mean it is not working. Often we have been programmed to be onions and heal in layers. Be receptive to healing all at once. Patience in waiting for Divine Timing is often a hard lesson.

Uncontrollable shaking during or after a session is a great thing. I have had this happen in every type of living being I have worked on. When I start to release, I shake enough to make people think I am having a seizure. There is a Religious Building that has a massive healing vortex in the center of it. I love to go and lay in the vortex in the basement. Often people come up to check on me, failing around on the floor like a fish. They think I am in distress, but no, I am in bliss. I believe this happens because the session causes the release of things that are no longer needed which raises the energy body's vibration, so the physical body shakes to catch up. It is ok if you or the intended receiver do not notice this shaking, because it may be still doing it at some other level.

Help the body detox and release. A lot of things are stirred up during the process, and I do not want them to land someplace within the body. So just like getting a massage, drink more water. Soak feet or body in hot Epsom salt or combination of sea salt and baking soda. Use ionic foot detox or sauna if available. Go hug a tree or re connect to your roots in whatever way works for you. If doing anonymous distant healing, you could do these yourself and possibly add the intent during the session to help the receiver detox and release.

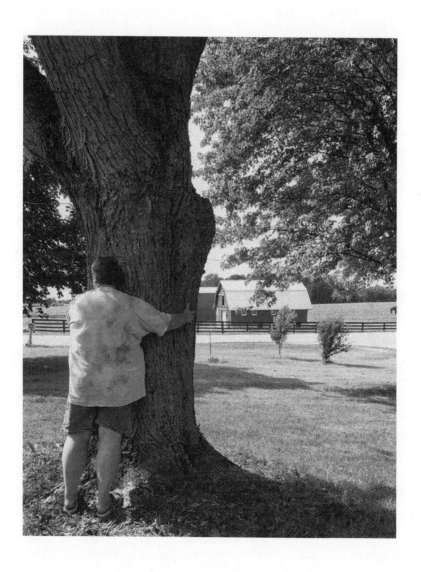

Tools

Helpful Tools you may Want in your Tool Box

DAILY CONNECTION

As often as you can, reconnect with your "Source" in whatever way works for you. I will use the word Source as to not offend anyone for what is their root truth, God, Love, Light, Spirit, Bubba, Creator, Divine, etc. I believe that "Source" is too large to be placed into one name. COEXIST in PEACE…..

"Spirit" (my Guides, Angels, Inner Voice, Creator, etc.) has given me a Native American 7 direction very brief ceremony. Often this can be done in less than a minute. Sometimes I do not know what direction East is for my starting point. That is when I will close my eyes, spin slowly in a circle until I feel or hear stop for a good starting point.

Stand facing East / Where the Sun rises from, in a vortex or favorite spot if possible, but where ever will work. If not in a favorite place in reality, close eyes and mentally go there. I place my hands outstretched palms up. I give love and great gratitude, during which I am pulled forward. I ask, often mentally, for all that is needed to walk in balance for this day, during which I am pushed backward. When I can stand straight, I turn right a quarter turn (90 degrees), repeat for South. Turn right a quarter turn, repeat for West / where the sun sets. Turn right a quarter turn, repeat for North. Aim hands, face and eyes to the ground, grow or reconnect the roots from your body into the center of Mother Earth. Release all things that no longer serve your highest good through those roots back into Mother Earth. Repeat the process of giving love, great gratitude and asking for balance. Aim hands, face and eyes to above, open up your crown chakra and reconnect with all great things above that dwells in Father Sky. Repeat the process. Put hands on the abdomen, repeat for the Great Mystery Within and the Body Temple where Source / Creator / God / Divine are invited to live. Take a moment to be in that space thoroughly Loved, Supported, Connected and in Balance.

Repeat as needed.

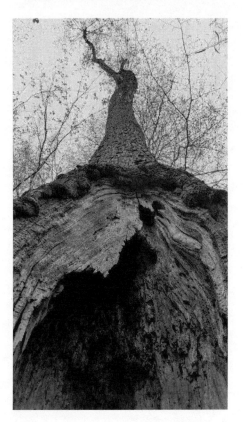

REIKI

Reiki is pronounced: Ray as in ray of light and Key as key to unlocking a door. Rei means spiritual wisdom, ki means energy, and so Reiki means spiritual energy. Reiki is not a religion even though it may or may not be one of the ways Jesus healed others. Reiki is a gentle, non-invasive healing practice that channels Universal energy to alleviate physical and emotional pain. Reiki training is passed down from Reiki Master / Teachers to students via instruction and Attunements. An Attunement is a ceremony that opens up energetic pathways in the body. Dr. Mikao Usui Original Five Principles are: Just for today I will give thanks for my many blessings. Just for today, I will not worry. Just for today, I will not be angry. Just for today, I will do my work honestly. Just for today, I will be kind to my neighbor and every living thing. A more positive affirmation form: Just for today, I will give thanks for my many blessings. Just for today, I will look at the positive. Just for today, I will deal with anger appropriately. Just for today, I will do my work honestly. Just for today, I will be kind to everyone and everything.

While I was at Veterinary Acupuncture School, one of the teachers, gave a very short description of Reiki. I believe he said, "you open up the Crown / top of your head to funnel in Universal Energy. You grow roots out of your feet to ground into the Earth." That was all I needed for my cellular memory to turn on and after that my hand would get hot while I worked. I was good with that for many years until a Reiki teacher came to me. His way was to do four treatments for you and then do an attunement. I still do it this way, because I feel the body is ready to receive the attunement.

I love to have Reiki as the base of Energy Healing because the Attunement hardwires the body to use Universal energy instead of Life force energy. The healer is not as drained. I also have said, that at some point in my life, I may need my life force energy and I don't want the tank to be empty. Attunements heighten the receiver's gifts / talents. Attunements help wash away the garbage from the receiver's life, sometimes faster than wanted. I have been taught that the Universe pays forward the Attunement receiver by clearing Karma. I wish everyone was Attuned, what a wonderful world it would be......

My daughter had her first Reiki Attunement at age 5. She would fall asleep each night with her hands on her first dog. I would also help her work on him at times while she was awake. He went from having all of the signs of stomach cancer to back to normal very quickly. She had not yet been programmed that cancer is incurable....

Reiki books I use and recommend to others, listed from most loved: The Reiki Healing Bible, Janet Green; Reiki for Dummies, Nina L. Paul, PhD; Reiki Hands That Heal, Joyce J. Morris, M.S., C.A.D.C., Reiki Master Teacher; Essential Reiki, A Complete Guide to an Ancient Healing Art, Diane Stein.

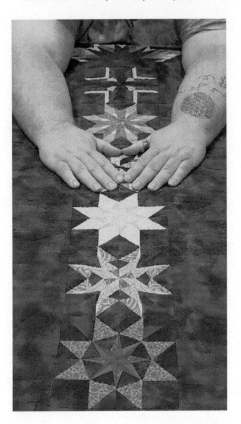

QUANTUM TOUCH

Quantum Touch uses life-force energy in hands-on and distant healing. Richard Gordon claims that the ability to heal is an inherent part of people's essential nature so that the ability to help heal each other is automatically built into everyone's system. Basic Quantum-Touch breathing techniques, body awareness meditations, and hand positions can be learned and applied very quickly.

Universe sent about ten messages about Quantum Touch in a two week period, before I said yes, I would learn it (9/7/2008) and then teach it. I love that it can increase the energy flowing from wherever you are. I love that it offers people that want to do Energy Healing but scared of "Reiki for Religious Beliefs" a way to get started. What my clients and patients love the most from my Quantum Touch training, is that I can move bones and other body parts with energy. Rolling ribs back into place and fixing pelvis rotation with a very light touch are some of my most favorite Random Acts of Healing to people I just meet.

After combining Reiki and Quantum Touch, there would be a noticeable decrease in size in many masses after I had laid hands on them for some time. There was one old black dog who had a tumor in her throat that would grow so large that she could not eat or drink. The owner total loved this dog but was on a very limited income. "Mom" would bring her in and I would sit on the floor with her with my hand on her throat for an hour. At the end of the treatment, the mass would be smaller. She would go home and be able to eat and drink once again. This cycle was repeated many times and probably add a year or so to their time together.

Quantum Touch, The Power to Heal, Richard Gordon, https://quantumtouch.com/

AWESOMENESS CUBED NESTING DOLLS TECHNIQUE

Spirit has given me this nesting doll technique to magnify the healing energy significantly for distant work. I cup my hands together, sometimes with arms crossed at the wrist but often not. I place the intended receiver or area of focus within my hands. When this feels complete, I place another mini-me with cupped hands holding the same thing inside of my hands also. I repeat this process or just ask that it continues infinitely. Sometimes I will expand in the same way but bigger than myself.

MUSCLE RESPONSE TESTING (MRT) / APPLIED KINESIOLOGY

Muscle Response Testing (also known as Applied Kinesiology) is a practice that is used to tap into the subconscious mind to answer questions about physical, mental, and emotional well-being. It's a noninvasive method that can be used to determine the underlying causes of ailments and afflictions an individual might be suffering from, identifying everything from nutritional needs to Trapped Emotions. I teach this to many of my clients to help empower them to make better choices for themselves and loved ones.

I learned MRT in California while attending a Veterinary Nambudripad Allergy Elimination Technique (NAET) Course. I learned there how to use the arm of a seragot, if yes or strong the arm would not move. If the response was no or weak the arm would easily be moved. It did not take me long to realize my clients in this small rural area where not going to go for this. So I quickly became skilled in the finger flick method. This is my favorite way to do MRT without anyone possibly knowing it is being done. You put your middle or ring finger just inside of your thumb, just like you would be going to flick something away. For me, a strong or yes response the hand stays in the same position. A weak or no response for me the middle or ring finger flies open. Almost from the beginning if it is a "bad allergy" I will get nauseous while testing. I have been doing MRT so much, a long time ago I was able to feel a switch inside my brain open or close. My clients surely can't see what's going on in my brain; winner, winner.

There are many ways to do MRT. My favorite one to teach to people who have never done it before is the Standing MRT. Stand up with your feet flat or on the balls of your feet if flat doesn't work for you. Ask your body to give you a yes. What does your body do? Sometimes it is better to have someone else watch you too let you know what it is doing. Often people will lend forward. Then ask your body to give you a No. What does your body do? Often people will lend backward. Your movement could be different which could be because of your polarity, but for whatever reason that's OK. If you get no movement, then picture yourself standing in a doorway with the best feast in front of you and the worst ever garbage dump behind you and repeat the process. Once you have your body's yes and no, then any yes / no question can be asked. Would this be helpful? Am I or my loved one allergic to this? Should I eat this? etc. The more you practice, the easier it becomes.

DOWSING

Dowsing is best known for a way to find underground water. A person would walk around while holding a y shaped stick or two bent rods until they moved to indicate where the intended searched object was located. This is still true today, but your imagination is the only thing that limits the intended search object. The same fundamental principle can be done with a pendulum, necklace, threaded needle, bobber, or dowsing rods. When using one you can find out the sex of the unborn child, get simple yes/no questions answered, detailed answers while using a chart at the same time, or clearing with adding, removing, or balancing energies and much more.

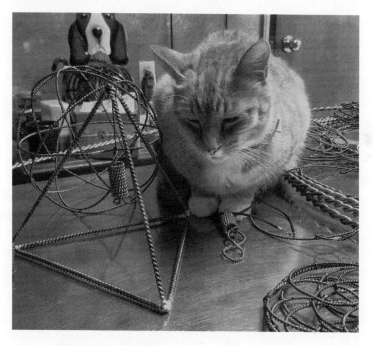

Dr. Frank using his first copper pendulum

I hosted a class with Raymon Grace in October 2010. He had said start by asking your dowsing tool for a yes, then no, then cleaning by adding, and then clearing by removing. If it does not move, you swing it to teach it what you want. He also said that, while dowsing the brain operates in all brain frequencies at the same time. He explained that this makes it easier and faster to get energetic changes done while dowsing. So feel free to hold your favorite dowsing tool while going through any of my projects and just let it fly without really needing to understand what is happening at all levels.

I would also like to recommend, that whenever dowsing demand your responses come only from Love, Light, Source, etc. This could be easily done by saying "in the name of the Light", (Lynn Grabhorn) at least until you are sure you can feel the source is pure.

Shortly after my weekend with Raymon Grace is when my very first healing list was written. Raymon had prompted us to do projects and this was one of mine. He helped me see that everything is energy and I now knew how to change it for the better.

Recommend Dowsing Teachers: Raymon Grace, http://www.raymongrace.us/; Jean Haner, " Clear Home, Clear Heart, Learn To Clear The Energy Of People & Places", https://www.jeanhaner.com/; Marie Diamond, http://www.mariediamond.com/.

COMPASSION KEY

Edward Mannix's Compassion Key is a simple yet powerful system for healing the inner child and clearing karmic imprints and distortions. People who work with The Compassion Key often report miracles in their financial life, relationships and health, as well as greater purpose alignment and feelings of lightness, relief and coming home to their true self. The Compassion Key shortcut technique can have rapid, long-lasting results. I am so sorry......

I was lead to Edward Mannix from Richard Gordon through a web call. As I listen to the way, Edward Facilitated this Compassion Key shortcut technique to others my brain was in panic mode. Here he was saying he was Sorry for all these bad things. So in my mind, he was not taking full acceptance of the problem without love, so he was going just to manifest more of the bad. I took a couple of deep breaths, grounded, my guides said it was just a tool go with it, my heart opened up, and then I felt wave after wave of karmic and negative energy release from my energy field. I was able to do several more web calls with Edward. During one of them, I was one of the callers to go through the process myself first hand just as I had seen in my dream the night before. I went through his Light Workers Accelerator course. I was one of the first 12 around the world to be in Edward Mannix's Compassion Key Certification Program. Edward and I often disagreed about the effectiveness of sorry vs. love during this program. But during our last call, I read my 9 pages of Compassion Key Statements with sorry and love both used. Edward literally had to pick himself off the floor after I was done and he said he could feel the different energies in the two wording...

My fastest Compassion Key Success story is of me and my "Home". I was working on a family friend at 11 am when she asked me "how was Poppers (my Father) doing?". I replied he was trying to sell the house I had lived at while in high school, so I was feeling homeless. I then said someone had committed suicide in my bed, so I did not ever want to stay there again. I internally went through Compassion Key Statements about that. At 7 pm that same night, my Father left a message, he had sold the house that afternoon, received the full cash payment before closing, and the lawyer could not believe it.

My most favorite Compassion Key Success Story also involves Poppers. I had gone to a "Light Expo" where so many strange things had occurred. I had a Spirit Painting done, and she said, I had to make things right with my father. I was not aware there was anything wrong... So once I got home, before going into the house with all of this new baggage, I sat on my bench next to the enormous vortex. I did Compassion Key Statements for everything strange over the weekend and did all that I could come up with for Poppers and me. There was a great love for him, but he is a workaholic. All of our vacations included work of some sort. He was often too busy to reach out to me. Later that day he called me. He started sending us Flowers for every occasion. He went on two fun only vacations within a month from my statements. He has taken us on fun vacations every year since then. He is still happily working at 77 years young. Do what you love and it is not a JOB. Blessed and Grateful we are...

Edward Mannix http://edwardmannix.com/
The Compassion Key https://compassionkey.com/

THE MOSES CODE

"I am that, I am."

I feel this statement helps remind us we are all one while at the same time calling acceptance to everything.

If I know what it is I want to address, I remove "that" and fill in the blank. I am _____, I am. I then repeat the statement with the opposite thing, because we carry every emotion or action within us at some level. So if sad were what I was working on, the statements would be: I am sad, I am. I am happy, I am.

I may not have all the information. The root cause of the problem is often unknown; it may be inherited or past life. In either case, I just keep repeating the statement and let inspiration and Universe figure out the details.

I watched a video on it, but there is a book by James F Twyman called "The Moses Code The Most Powerful Manifestation Tool in the History of the World".

HO'OPONOPONO

Ho'oponopono originated from Hawaii and means to make right. Essentially, it means to make it right with the ancestor or to make right with the people with whom you have relationships. Morrnah Nalamaku Simeona initially taught ho'oponopono. In 1983 she received a great honor by being designated as a living treasure of Hawaii. Haleaka

Hew Len Ph.D., a Hawaiian psychologist, and shamanic practitioner cured a complete ward of criminally insane patients – without ever seeing any of them. Dr. Hew Len would study an inmate's chart and then look within himself to see how he created that person's illness. As he improved himself using Ho'oponopono, the patient also improved. Dr. Joe Vitale heard about Dr. Hew Len and then later they created an online Ho'oponopono Course/Certification. http://www. hooponoponocertification.com/

HO'OPONOPONO SIMPLE STATEMENT: I Love You. I am Sorry. Please Forgive Me. Thank you.

HA Soul breathing, infusing Devine / Source, breathing into the four corners of the universe, endless beginnings, closes lots of physic doors…. Inhale, hold, exhale, pause for all equal lengths (10 counts) repeat 10 times. In the certification class, Dr. Hew Len said you could say "I love you" for each part and hold thumb and a finger together.

I have been inspired to inhale / I love you, hold / please forgive me, exhale / I am sorry, pause / thank you. I also move the thumb to the next finger after each cycle. I do include the invisible finger just past the little finger. Spirit told me to start using this finger for NAET treatments because each fingering runs energy through a different energy circuit in the body. There is an amazing amount of garbage carried in that invisible finger; I often am gagging with that one during NAET treatments. Two possible reasons it is needed is as the embryo's there is this extra finger that starts and then goes away and that inhabitants from the Pleiades have six fingers on each hand (I have been told by a man). I have found it tremendously helpful to do this before going to sleep and repeat if I can't fall back to sleep in the middle of the night.

I was referred to this course, took it, and passed in 4 days, 6/19/2017, while also working. It felt like I was coming home, to a place I did not know I missed. Some of the things that happen during those four days are even wild in my view. One of my canine patients looked blue only to me. I was craving tuna fish while watching one of the videos and about an hour later we could smell tuna fish around me without physical exposure to it. During my first HA, I sat on the bench in between my clinic and a vast healing vortex in the parking lot. An inspiration came that the empathic feeling within me maybe is where the Memory is stored within me that needs to be released for those I am working on. This was a major AHA moment for me. This made sense how if we are All One if I work on me, it will help you, and if you have problems that I am not a where of in myself, this empathic feeling just helped me locate and remove it for both of us. When I came back to this Earthly plane and opened my eyes, there was a pile of feathers and my Angel pendulum laying in front of me in the parking lot. I had not noticed them there before and did not even know my Angel pendulum had been missing because we had used it a couple of days before.

This is my essay I wrote for Ho'oponopono Certification:

> *"I would and already have since starting this program, help clients by taking the responsibility that whatever arises, the problem is a memory within me. I would continue cleaning, since now it is becoming a continuous process, but now with focus on what has come up. The cleaning refers to repeating the statement: "I love you, I am sorry, please forgive me, thank you," or even just I love you. By my cleaning the message can go down to my subconscious and then up to Divine, which can release Mana back down to remove that memory from me, my cells, and others including my client. On more intense issues I can incorporate HA a soul Breathing for infusing Divine as I am repeating the cleaning statement. Breath in – I love you, hold breath – I am sorry, Breath out – please forgive me, hold breath – thank you. Or once again I love you for breath moves to the 4 corners of the universe. I repeat this cycle 10 times to reach completion.*
>
> *Today I had a dog return for 3rd treatment that has disc problems. There has been great improvement with the*

combination of holistic treatments I have already been doing. However, today I was Inspired to add these new things to the mix. I placed my hands over the bad disc, closed my eyes, focused on bad disc/back pain memories in myself, and start HA. After the first 10 breath cycles my hands were getting very hot and the dogs back was feeling better. I repeated HA two more times with the same effect each time. When done the dogs back went from cat arched like to flat and the muscles were much more soft and pliable. The acupuncture needles were then place in and the dog was kicking them back out very quickly, were he has held on to them for days after previous treatments. Acupuncture needles will move out when the body is done with them, much like the indicator when cooking a turkey.

While watching these videos and learning this it has felt like coming home. So many very cool things have already happen in just the couple day since starting. I am very excited to see what else will come to clean and what inspiration will come. Thank you.

I love you.
I am sorry.
Please forgive me.
Thank you."

Spirit gave me a mixture of mostly doTERRA Essential Oils to be used as a Ho'oponopono Cleaning tool. I am a doTERRA Essential Oil consultant, www.mydoterra.com/sandrasnell. DoTERRA is my oil of choice because I can feel the energy, Every single doTERRA bottle I have touched is vibrating with amazing energy. I chose to raise vibration, rather than fight. Within a month of using doTERRA Essential Oils in my home and clinic, I received my Aha moment. The Essential Oils work far better than the herbs because of several things. First, they are easy to get them into the patient. I had given up on getting herbs into a cat. With the oils, you can put them on topically or if that's a problem diffuse them. But no one that I know of has stopped breathing the diffused oil. Though, my smart Orange Healing Cats, Frank and Jophiel, would knock over the diffuser placed in front of their cage when they had a head cold. Most importantly the Essential Oil contains the Life Force Energy of the plant, where the herb is from the old dried up carcass...

Months later, I was doing ho'oponopono all of the time. My "Darling" friend, who became certified in Ho'oponopono a couple of days after I did, and I had a little rough patch. She keeps telling me she was ho'oponopono our relationship. I was home alone, 8/9/17, sitting in my bedroom when the hall LED light started flashing in a disruptive pattern. I checked in with my guides, and all I heard was "dit, dit, dit, dot, dot, dot" as in Morse code. I just let it flash until I left the upstairs, then I turned it off for concern of fire. The next day, my daughter turned this light back on while I was sitting in my bedroom. She was scared out of her mind, came running over to me for protection, and then recorded it. She sent it straight to Darling, who kept saying it was Morse code also. The next day, Darling deciphered the video which contained the complete loop of ho'oponopono statement starting from the last word. "You Love You I am Sorry Please Forgive Me Thank"

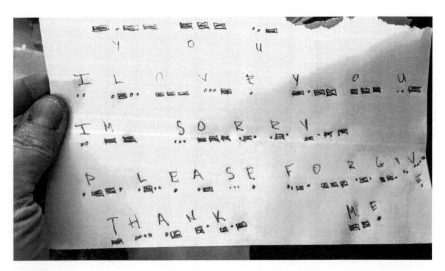

After adding Ho'oponopono and sometimes HA to my hands on treatments, I have felt masses shrink within my hands on man and beast. Some of the masses I can surround with my right hand have become unpalatable in minutes. I now have to remember to have the client feel it before, and after I focus on a mass, so they can appreciate what is possible and happening right in front of them.

COMBINING TOOLS

Spirit has inspired combining many of these tools. This is just a couple of examples.

DR. SANDRA SNELL'S HO'OPONOPONO EXPANDED STATEMENT on 1/15/18 (Moses Code & Doreen Virtue) I am That, I am. (or, I am _____, I am.) I Love You. I am Sorry. Please Forgive Me. Thank You. I release everything but the lessons and the LOVE. I Believe in Miracles. I Believe in You. I Believe in Me. God Bless You.

During a reiki session in April of 2018, Spirit explained that combining the Moses Code, Ho'oponopono and the Doreen Virtue sentence brings in the cubed power to the awesomeness...

On 7/25/2018 I had a issue at home. I sat with pendulum in hand read through many of the following projects, HA, followed Spirit and Channeled. When I felt It was complete, I looked up and was given inspiration. I connected my necklace I used as a pendulum to a wind chime and aimed a large fan at it. So it could continue spinning and raising vibration various ways. I asked my Angels to continue working. I followed my HEART while Prayer Warrioring...

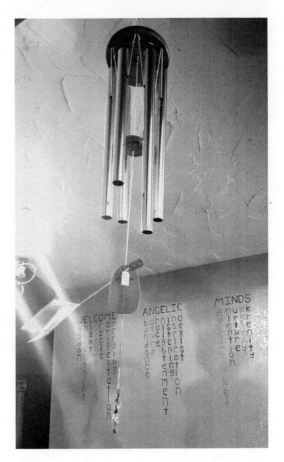

Combine them as you are led.

On 7/16/18 Megan Lyon's, Pre Vet Shadow, and I did a Reiki session on Megan's Mother. I had asked Megan to do Access Bars and Read through Project #10 (both are explained later in this book). Megan had been inspired to add the following to her readings. And so it is.

I believe in Miracles.
I believe in You.
I believe in Me.
I believe in Us.
I believe in We.
I believe in the Creator's
Love and Prosperity.
God Bless You and Me.

Projects

These are my inspired projects mostly in the order as given to me. As I learned and grew they would be tweaked or a whole new method would take form. Each Project is like a snapshot of where I was at that time in my Healing Path. To me, they get stronger as they get higher up in order.

I took my Veterinary Oath very seriously. Especially, Do no harm!!! As far as Spirit has informed me, none of my projects will cause harm. The benefits far outweigh any potential negative effects. These perceive negative effects may be needed for growth. Doors may be opened that were not before. HA breathing explained in Tools: Ho'oponopono should close them. If different things keep coming up in dreams and life, this could be Universe saying "Hi" this needs to be addressed.

Spirit is pushing me to hand all of these tools to you. So you can pick and chose what is right for you while you are doing your Prayer Warrioring at that time and space. By having so many, also hopefully helps you see how you can change things up to make it fit for whatever is needed at the time.

The way you can use them is only limited by your imagination. I have used them as a prayer. I have dowsed while saying them. I have said them alone. I have said them on the phone. I have said them to large groups holding hands around a vortex. I have read them out loud. I have read them only in my head and heart. I have used them during Energy Healing Sessions. I have used them in Ceremonies. I have had clients repeat them back to me. I have spoken them in Tongues. I have sang their essence in many songs. I have said them on a plane. I have said them on a boat. I have said them in a cave. I have said them on a horse. I would say them eating Green Eggs and Ham. I would say them anywhere. I would say them with anyone. I am Sand, Sand I am.

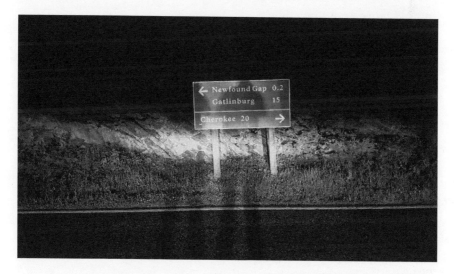

One of the following Projects was done while
crossing over the Smoky Mountains.
Only one Human was standing in front of vehicle
taking this picture on the return trip.

PROJECT # 1

SNELL DOWSING HEALING
GUIDE 11/3/2010

The initial intent is to direct this energy to _____, their family, animals, home, work, and projects.

All bodies including physical, mental, emotional, spiritual, light, and sound bodies are to be addressed.

Increase ability to forgive self, others, and Divine / Source.

Remove negative entities, forces, poltergeist, non beneficial E. T, s.

Bring soul to this dimension and fix fragmentations of the soul. Soul becomes whole, healed, complete, grounded, and compatible with body and self.

Increase patient's desire for improvement and decrease their resistance to your help.

Adjust the surface tension of water to eliminate the non-beneficial memory of water in the body of the traumas of this life and past lives. (negative cellular memory)

Activate the genes that need to activated. Deactivate the genes that need to be deactivated.

FORGIVE, TRANSMUTE, RELEASE / REMOVE / REDUCE / NEUTRALIZE NON BENEFICIAL EFFECTS

Negative energetic patterns, negative patterns of attraction, and negative thought forms, Curses, hexes, spells, black magic, witchcraft, bad medicine, attachments, hooks, daggers.

Stress of all kinds including geographic (water veins), Electromagnetic, A. C. current, sonar, Non-beneficial Spirit Guides, archetypes, psychic chords, toxic chords, programming / brainwashing, Negative karmic influences, Old vows or agreements including poverty, chastity, obedience, loyalty, suffering, etc.

Effect of heritage, culture & religion of ancestors.

Belief, thought & memories including inherited, self-imposed or by association.

All forms of repression and imprisonment including self-imposed.

Self-sabotage, self-destruct, self-hate, & self-punishment mental programs.

Spirits of victimization, co-dependency, disease, and emotions such as anger, greed, grief, unworthiness, doubt, shame, guilt, and fear including fear of success and fear of failure.

Miasmas, disease processes, addictions, excess body fat, non-beneficial bacteria, viruses, fungus, parasites, diabetes, allergies, sensitivities,

All chemical, biological, & radiological pollutants of water / body.

Hertz frequency effect on people and animals.

BALANCE / IDEAL LEVEL:

Universal energy - polarity, aura / clear holes, pH, body chemistry, metabolism.

Body senses including hearing, vision, taste, touch, and smell.

Body systems including matrix, lymphatic, nervous, respiratory, digestive, endocrine, urinary, circulatory, dermatological, hematological, etc.

Glands Including hypothalamus, pineal, thyroid, adrenal, etc.

Hormones including serotonin, noradrenaline, melatonin, etc.

Brain chemistry, brain blood flow, and right and left hemispheres.

Command Center including messages from the brain to the body (stroke).

Red and white blood cells, lithium, and amino acids.

Chakras, assemblage point, hara line, electrons.

To ideal body weight & size.

Light body & Sound body.

ADD / INCREASE

Energy level.

Body Frequency.

Strength of Nature Spirits, Guides, Angels, Magical Beings.

Compatibility and Communication with all beneficial guides (yours and others).

Connection with Divine / Source / true higher self / Mother Earth.

Degree of feeling wanted at birth and always.

Compatibility of body cells / spin of the cells, beneficial bacteria.

Activate cetyl - myristoleate (natural lubricant of the body).

Your body's desire to live, whole and each organ.

Your body's alignment with your original blueprint.

Body's ability to stay in alignment and ability to fix itself as needed.

Our ability to observe ourselves and knowledge, ability, and strength to make it right.

Positive Spirits including love, freedom, prosperity, perfect health, peace, joy, harmony, abundance, romance, passion, and sex (if age appropriate), etc.

Reprogram our body that anything we want to consume is good or neutral for us.

LAST STEP:

REBOOT THE BODY COMPUTER TO THE IDEAL SETTING

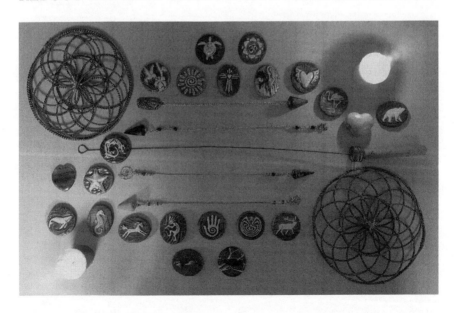

PROJECT # 2

SNELL LOVE DECLARATIONS 10/17/2015

I love you even though you may sometimes forget to "Fear Not" which is in the Bible 365 times.

I love you even though all of your bodies including your Physical, Emotional, Mental, Spiritual, Light and Sound bodies may not always have optimal ability to forgive yourself, forgive others, forgive Divine / Source and then transmute and release all things that do not resonate with your highest interest and good.

I love you even though you may have been adversely affected by negative entities, Demonic Kings and / or Forces, Poltergeist, non-beneficial E.T.s, negative energetic patterns, negative patterns of attractions, curses, hexes, spells, black magic, witchcraft, bad medicine, negative thought forms, attachments, hooks, or daggers.

I love you even though your Soul may be fragmented and not always in the current dimension of your body.

I love you even though your Soul may not always be whole, healed, complete, grounded, and compatible with self and others.

I love you even though you may not always have the highest desire for improvement.

I love you even though you may not always have the least resistance to help, heal, change and improve.

I love you even though the surface tension of water within your body is not always ideal to painlessly eliminate all non-beneficial memories of trauma and all negative cellular memory of this life and past lives.

I love you even though you may have trouble returning to Love, Balance, Wisdom, Self, and Source.

I love you even though you may have forgotten how to open Heaven and Enter.

I love you even though you do not return to your drawer in the Great Hall of the Akashic Records to retrieve missing Soul pieces and re-read your Soul purpose as often as needed.

I love you even though, you didn't receive the entire miracle all at once.

I love you even though you couldn't fix all parts of your life.

I love you even though you couldn't have what you want.

I love you even though you couldn't experience the joy of completion.

I love you even though you may feel trapped in an imperfect life.

I love you even though you may feel discounted from Source.

I love you even though you have trouble shining your Light and sharing your gifts fully.

I love you even though you may have been ridiculed, banished, exiled, tortured, buried alive and / or possibly killed for being the authentic you and Shining your Light and Powers in the past.

I love you even though you and others cannot always recognize, treat, and accept the great true light being that you are.

I love you even though you and others do not love and treat you as you need and or want.

I love you even though you may be sad.

I love you even though you may be angry.

I love you even though you may have been hurt, betrayed, stabbed in the back, raped or killed on some level.

I love you even though you may have been abandoned or felt all alone.

I love you even though you were programmed and under the illusion when loved ones leave this plane, that we have lost our connection with them.

I love you even though you do not always relate to ones that have passed as the brilliant Soul / energy source they are.

I love you even though you were not always able to save others or self.

I love you even though you miss the physical accepts of lost love.

I love you even though there may be broken promises by self and others.

I love you even though more memories could not be made or remembered.

I love you even though you may not feel worthy of all the wonderful things you deserved and was bestowed on to you from Source.

I love you even though you sometimes have trouble learning the lessons, so you have to be re-exposed to the "problem" repeatedly.

I love you even though you may keep getting blocks on your path, including self-imposed and self- sabotage.

I love you even though you may feel you need to carry and heal the world all on your own.

I love you even though your ability to think and follow your own truth often threatens and scares others.

I love you even though you have trouble just being one of the subservient masses or herds patiently following the others even if you are being lead to slaughter.

I love you even though you're important things are not always valued by others.

I love you even though others may like to treat you poorly.

I love you even though you have given so much of your time, energy, emotion, and power away to someone else.

I love you even more because you keep raising your vibration / searching for enlightenment even though it often means loved ones leave and / or are not comfortable being around you anymore.

I love you even though you felt, learned, and wasted so much energy on the illusion of your coping system to rectify past trauma.

I love you even though you may not always be able to follow / have your "Having It All Statement."

I love you even though you may still have to work and not at financial freedom yet.

MOST COMPATIBLE SOUL MATE

I love you even more because your Self Love is not always perfect.

I love you even though you may sometimes forget you are made from love and are worthy of love.

I love you even though you may forget you are perfect just the way you are.

I love you even though you may have trouble finding and keeping your most compatible Soul Mate.

I love you even though you may not always remember you can clear all the blocks between you and your most compatible Soul Mate.

I love you even though you may not always feel deserving of receiving your most compatible Soul Mate.

I love you even though your most compatible Soul Mate is in mourning or term oil of their own and may not have found you yet.

I love you even though you may sometimes forget that you do not have to heal your most compatible Soul Mate because they can do it themselves.

I love you even though you may sometimes forget "the person you're meant to be with will never have to be chased, begged, or give an ultimatum." (Mandy Hale)

BALANCE / IDEAL

I love you even though you may not have optimal flow and amount of Universal Energy, polarity, Soul, and aura.

I love you even though you may have holes in your Soul and aura.

I love you even though you may not have optimal pH of body, intake, and output.

I love you even though you may not have optimal metabolism, body and brain chemistry.

I love you even though you may not have optimal performance and balance of all body systems, hormones, glands, amino acids, electrons, senses, chakras, meridians, and body forms.

I love you even though you have not been able to automatically reset all of your Allowing Meter to ideal for Love, Abundance, Freedom, Vitality, happiness, ease, pleasure, self-worth, self-love, divine connections, body shape and weight and all other meters that do not resonate with your highest good.

I love you even though your body may not be completely balanced in all ways and forms.

I love you even though parts of your body may not be equally feeling and sharing the love and healing.

REMOVE / REDUCE

I love you even though you may have been negatively affected by your heritage and lineage from this life and past lives.

I love you even though you may have been negatively affected by Archival types, beliefs, culture, karmic influences, society, politics, and religion of self and ancestors.

I love you even though you may have been negatively affected by old vows or agreements such as poverty, chastity, obedience, loyalty, suffering, etc.

I love you even though you may have been negatively affected by beliefs, thoughts and memories be it inherited, self-imposed, or by association.

I love you even though you may have been negatively affected by Geographic Stresses and electromagnetic fields, such as water veins, Hertz frequencies, A-C current, and sonar.

I love you even though you may have been negatively affected by Spirits of victimization, codependency, diseases, and attachment such as past trauma.

I love you even though you may have been negatively affected by strong emotions such as fear, anger, greed, grief, unworthiness, doubt, shame, sadness, depression, and guilt including of success and failure.

I love you even though you may have been negatively affected by psychic chords, toxic chords, and any other connections to people, places, and things not for your highest good.

I love you even though you may have been negatively affected by all forms of repression and imprisonment including those self-imposed.

I love you even though you may have been negatively affected by miasmas, disease processes, diagnosis cancer, yeast, addictions, non-beneficial bacteria, viruses, fungi, parasites, allergies, sensitivities, pesticides, GMOs and heavy metals.

I love you even though you may have been negatively affected by all pollutants including chemical, biological, and radiological.

I love you even though you may have been negatively affected by non-beneficial Spirit Guides, teachers, leaders, friends, and relatives.

I love you even though you may have been negatively affected by implants of all types.

I love you even though you may have been adversely affected by all forms of programming including brainwashing.

I love you even though you may sometime believe you need to suffer in life and relationships.

I love you even though all of your limiting beliefs have not been detected and destroyed.

I love you even though limitations may not have been destroyed, dissolved, blown up and away.

I love you even though others may not see, feel or honor the drama free bubble around you.

I love you even though unstable people keep having to play out the drama in front of you to prove themselves or something.

I love you even though you may sometimes forget that just because some people are fueled by drama, it doesn't mean you have to attend the performance.

I love you even though you may have felt you had limited life choices.

I love you even though you may have to do things you do not want to do or doesn't seem to follow your soul purpose.

I love you even though patience can be a hard lesson about Divine timing.

I love you even though you may have to deal with others that don't understand you.

I love you even though you do not have perfect knowledge / vision on this side of the veil.

I love you even though you may have trouble completely forgiving Devine / Source, others, and Self.

ADD/INCREASE

I love you even though you may not always have felt wanted, loved and enough.

I love you even though your joy and purpose may be so hidden.

I love you even though you may not always have optimal energy level or body frequency.

I love you even though you may not always have optimal strength, connection, and compatibility with your True Self, Devine / Source,

Spirit Guides, Angels, Nature Spirits, Animal Totems, and Magical Beings.

I love you even though you may not always have optimal compatibility of body cells and spin of the cells.

I love you even though you may not always have an optimal body and soul alignment with your original Blueprint.

I love you even though you may not always have optimal desire to live for the whole body, each organ, and each cell.

I love you even though you may not always have optimal connections with Positive Spirits such as Love, Freedom, Prosperity, Perfect Health, Peace, Joy, Harmony, Abundance, Passion, Romance, and Sex (if age appropriate).

I love you even though you may not always have optimal positive patterns of attraction for things that help your highest good such as freedom, prosperity, optimal relationships including with your most compatible Soul Mate.

I love you even though you may not always have optimal amounts of beneficial bacteria.

I love you even though you may not always have optimal settings on all of your Allowing Meters.

I love you even though you may not always have optimal chemistry and communication throughout the entire body.

I love you even though you may not always have the optimal balance between the para-sympatric and sympatric nervous systems.

I love you even though you may not always have optimal absorption of the appropriate nutrients of all food and drink consumed to maintain ideal size and weight and chemistry.

I love you even though you may not always have the optimal knowledge, desire and ability to eat and drink only things that are good for you.

I love you even though you may not always have the ability to reprogram your body so that anything you do consume is right for you.

I love you even though you may not always have optimal levels of natural body lubrication.

I love you even though you may not always have optimal structural and spiritual alignment and the ability to autocorrect as needed.

I love you even though you may not always have the optimal ability to observe yourselves and knowledge, skill, and strength to make it right.

I love you even though you may not always remember your value doesn't decrease based on someone's inability to see your worth.

I love you even though you may not always remember that your words have power and ability to use them wisely. Therefore, eliminate bad and limiting self-talk and thought.

I love you even though you may not always have the optimal vision of time and space.

I love you even though you may not always have optimal connection or recall of your higher purpose or the big picture.

I love you even though you may not always have the optimal knowledge, ability, and strength on how best to serve self, others, and the planet.

I love you even though you may not always have an optimal passion for life.

I love you even though you may not always have an optimal connection and knowledge for painless downloads.

I love you even though you may not always have optimal recall and execution of all Universal Laws and Symbols.

I love you even though you sometimes may forget the Law of Attraction and maybe focusing on things you may not really want.

I love you even though you may not always have optimal knowledge and execution of all Laws of Creation and any other Laws our higher self must follow.

I love you even though if you only focus on the problem, you might miss the easy solution.

I love you even though you may not always able to automatically reset the body computer to ideal.

I love you even though you may not always have optimal faith.

I love you even though you may not always have optimal Love, courage, strength, knowledge, and wisdom in all things.

I love you even though you may struggle to allow the joy and happiness into your life.

I love you even though you may not always remember and believe you deserve lightness, love, happiness, peace, harmony, and joy in your day to day life.

I love you even though you don't always attract what you expect, reflect what you desire, become what you respect, or mirror what you admire.

I love you even though you are not always surrounded with the dreamers and the doers, the thinks, but most of all, surround yourself with those who see the greatness within you, even when you don't see it yourself.

I love you even though not all your friends help you to find important things when you have lost them…. Your smile, your hope, and your courage.

I love you even though you may have forgotten passion isn't about finding the purpose for others in one's path, but letting your focus be on purpose and passion will be found.

I love you even though you may have been under the illusion that "the truth that sets one free isn't the truth that other ones see, but the truth that one confronts within yourself."

I love you even though you may not always be able to be in harmony with your spirit which is like a flowing river. You go where you will without pretense and arrives at your destination prepared to be yourself and only yourself. (Maya Angelou)

I love you even more because you may not always remember that your heart knows the way and you may not have the strength, knowledge, and ability to run in that direction. (Rumi)

I love you even though you may suffer from "PTSD - Post-Traumatic Sandy Disease."

OR THE SHORT FORM

I LOVE YOU EVEN MORE WHEN OTHERS MAY NOT ACCEPT LOVE IS YOUR RELIGION.
I LOVE YOU EVEN MORE WHEN YOU MAY NOT KNOW and REMEMBER IT.
I LOVE YOU EVEN WHEN YOU ARE NOT OVERFLOWING WITH SELF LOVE!!!
I LOVE YOU EVEN THOUGH YOU MAY BE AFRAID and PROGRAMMED NOT TO BE ABLE TO
- REMEMBER OR SEE YOUR TRUE SELF.
-EXPRESS YOUR LOVE TO OTHERS.
-BE ABLE TO LOVE YOURSELF.

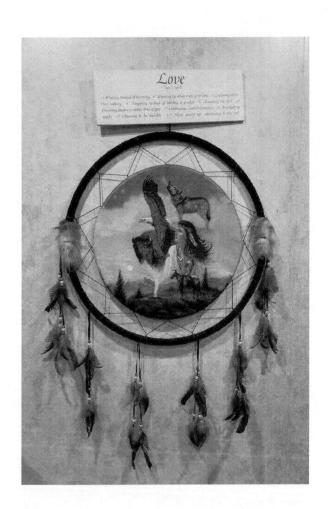

PROJECT # 3

SNELL LOVE DECLARATIONS 2/20/2016

I love you even more because you are still here.

I love you even though you may sometimes forget to "Fear Not" which is in the Bible 365 times.

I Love you even though all of your bodies including your Physical, Emotional, Mental, Spiritual, Light and Sound bodies may not always have optimal ability to forgive yourself, forgive others, forgive Divine / Source and then transmute and release all things that do not resonate with your highest interest and good.

I love you even though you may have been adversely affected by negative entities, Demonic Kings and/or Forces, Poltergeist, non-beneficial E.T.s, negative energetic patterns, negative patterns of attractions, curses, hexes, spells, black magic, witchcraft, bad medicine, negative thought forms, attachments, hooks, or daggers.

I love you even though your Soul may be fragmented and not always in the current dimension of your body.

I love you even though your Soul may not always be whole, healed, complete, grounded, and compatible with self and others.

I love you even though you may not always have the highest desire for improvement.

I love you even though you may not always have the least resistance to help, heal, change and improve.

I love you even though the surface tension of water within your body is not always ideal to painlessly eliminate all non-beneficial memories of trauma and all negative cellular memory of this life and past lives.

I love you even though you may or may not be a Lightworker.

I love you even though you may have trouble returning to Love, Balance, Wisdom, Self, and Source.

I love you even though you may have forgotten how to open Heaven and Enter.

I love you even though you do not return to your drawer in the Great Hall of the Akashic Records to retrieve missing Soul pieces and re-read your Soul purpose as often as needed.

I love you even though you didn't receive the entire miracle all at once.

I love you even though you couldn't always fix all parts of your life.

I love you even though you couldn't always have what you want.

I love you even though you couldn't always experience the joy of completion.

I love you even though you may feel trapped in an imperfect life.

I love you even though you may feel discounted from Source.

I love you even though you have trouble shining your Light and sharing your gifts fully.

I love you even more because you may have been ridiculed, banished, exiled, tortured, buried alive and / or possibly killed for being the authentic you and Shining your Light and Powers in the past.

I love you even though you and others cannot always recognize, treat, and accept the great true light being that you are.

I love you even though you and others do not love and treat you as you need and or want.

I love you, even more, when you are sad.

I love you, even more, when you are angry.

I love you even though you may have been hurt, betrayed, stabbed in the back, raped or killed on some level.

I love you even though you may have been abandoned or felt all alone.

I love you even though you were programmed and under the illusion when loved ones leave this plane, that we have lost our connection with them.

I love you even though you do not always relate to ones that have passed as the brilliant soul / energy source they are.

I love you even though you were not always able to save others or self.

I love you even though you miss the physical accepts of lost love.

I love you even though there may have been broken promises.

I love you even though more memories could not be made or remembered.

I love you even though you may not feel worthy of all the wonderful things you deserved and was bestowed on to you by Divine.

I love you even though you may be affected by outside influence.

I love you even though you may be a collector of other people stuff.

I love you even though you may have malaise to God / Source.

I love you, even more, when you sometimes have trouble learning the lessons, so you have to be re-exposed to the "problem" repeatedly.

I love you even though you keep getting blocks on your path, including self-imposed and self- sabotage.

I love you even more because often you feel you need to carry and heal the world all on your own.

I love you even more because often your ability to think and follow your truth threatens and scares others.

I love you even though you have trouble just being one of the subservient masses or herds patiently following the others even if you are being lead to slaughter.

I love you even though your important things are not always valued by others.

I love you even though others may like to treat you badly or worse.

I love you even though you have given so much of your time, energy, emotion, and power away to someone else.

I love you even more because you keep raising your vibration / searching for enlightenment even though it often means loved ones leave and are not comfortable being around you anymore.

I love you even though you felt, learned, and wasted so much energy on the illusion of your coping system to rectify past trauma.

I love you even though you may not always be able to follow / have your "Having It All Statement."

I love you even though you may still have to work because you're not at financial freedom yet.

I love you even though your primary need for Attachment may have over ridened your necessary need to be authentic.

I love you even though this pattern may have created a coping mechanism in you.

I love you even though this coping mechanism may have outrun its usefulness and may be causing disease.

I love you even though this possible disease may not as of yet totally opened you back up to your authentic self.

I love you even though all those you made Attachments with were not always safe or healthy.

I love you even though you are not always your most authentic self.

I love you even though you may forget that free will choice can even trump God / Source.

I love you even though you may forget to respect someone's choices for themselves.

I love you even though you may not remember to utilize all of your gifts.

I love you even though you may not know what all of your gifts are.

I love you even though you may forget to turn worries into prayers.

I love you even though you may have trouble forgiving and releasing everything but the lesson and the love.

I love you even though you may not always be acutely aware of your true feelings, and always follow your heart.

I love you even though you may not always notice signs from self, Source, Guides, Angels, and Universe.

I love you even though you may doubt you are always Enough!

MOST COMPATIBLE SOUL MATE

I love you even more because your Self Love is not always perfect.

I love you even though you may sometimes forget you are made from love and are worthy of love.

I love you even though you may forget you are perfect just the way you are.

I love you even though you may often have relationship problems and may not recognize and handle them correctly.

I love you even though you may have trouble finding and keeping your most compatible Soul Mate.

I love you even though you may not always remember you can clear all the blocks between you and your most compatible Soul Mate.

I love you even though you may not always feel deserving of receiving your most compatible Soul Mate.

I love you even though your most compatible Soul Mate is in mourning or term oil of their own and may not have found you yet.

I love you even though you may sometimes forget that you do not have to heal your most compatible Soul Mate because they can do it themselves.

I love you even though you may sometimes forget "the person you're meant to be with will never have to be chased, begged, or give an ultimatum." (Mandy Hale)

BALANCE / IDEAL

I love you even though you may not have optimal flow and amount of Universal Energy, polarity, and aura.

I love you even though you may have holes in your aura.

I love you even though you may not have optimal pH in body, intake, and output.

I love you even though you may not have optimal metabolism, body and brain chemistry.

I love you even though you may not have optimal performance and balance of all body systems, hormones, glands, amino acids, electrons, senses, chakras, and body forms.

I love you even though you have not been able to automatically reset all of your Allowing Meter to ideal for Love, Abundance, Freedom, Vitality, happiness, ease, pleasure, self-worth, self-love, Divine / Source connections, body shape and weight and all other meters that do not resonate with your highest good.

I love you even though your body may not be completely balanced in all ways and forms.

I love you even though parts of your body may not be equally feeling and sharing the love and healing.

REMOVE / REDUCE

I love you even though you may have been negatively affected by your heritage and lineage from this life and past lives.

I love you even though you may have been negatively affected by Archival types, beliefs, culture, karmic influences, society, politics, and religion of self and ancestors.

I love you even though you may have been negatively affected by old vows or agreements such as poverty, chastity, obedience, loyalty, suffering, etc.

I love you even though you may have been negatively affected by beliefs, thoughts, memories, and conflict be it inherited, self-imposed, or by association.

I love you even though you may have been negatively affected by Geographic Stresses and electromagnetic fields, such as water veins, Hertz frequencies, A-C current, and sonar.

I love you even though you may have been negatively affected by Spirits of victimization, codependency, diseases, and attachment such as past trauma.

I love you even more because you may be very sensitive to energy, chemicals, emotions, diseases, conflict, other people's opinions, etc.

I love you even though you may have been negatively affected by strong emotions such as fear, anger, greed, grief, unworthiness, doubt, shame, sadness, depression, and guilt.

I love you even though you may have been negatively affected by psychic chords, toxic chords, and any other connections to people, places, and things not for your highest good.

I love you even though you may have been negatively affected by all forms of repression and imprisonment including those self-imposed.

I love you even though you may have been negatively affected by miasmas, disease processes, diagnosis, cancer, yeast, addictions, non–beneficial bacteria, viruses, fungi, parasites, allergies, sensitivities, pesticides, GMOs and heavy metals.

I love you even though you may have been negatively affected by all pollutants including chemical, biological, and radiological.

I love you even though you may have been negatively affected by non-beneficial Spirit Guides, teachers, leaders, friends, and relatives.

I love you even though you may have been negatively affected by implants of all types.

I love you even though you may have been adversely affected by all forms of programming including brainwashing.

I love you even though you give unto overs for any reason, more than you give to yourself.

I love you even though your protective limits were not always in place or followed.

I love you even when you have to help expert victims.

I love you, even more, when that expert victim you helped is attacking you.

I love you even though everyone's definition of "emergency" is not the same.

I love you even though you may sometime believe you need to suffer in life and relationships.

I love you even though all of your limiting beliefs have not been detected and destroyed.

I love you even though limitations may not have been destroyed, dissolved, blown up and away.

I love you even though others may not see, feel or honor the drama free bubble around you.

I love you even though unstable people keep having to play out their drama in front of you.

I love you even though you may sometimes forget that just because some people are fueled by drama, it doesn't mean you have to attend the performance.

I love you even though you may have limited life choices.

I love you even though you may have felt you made the wrong choice.

I love you even though you may have to do things you do not want to do or doesn't seem to follow your soul purpose.

I love you even though patience can be the hard lesson about divine timing.

I love you even though you may have to deal with others that don't understand you.

I love you even though you do not have perfect knowledge / vision on this side of the veil.

I love you even though you may have trouble completely forgiving Divine / Source, others, and Self.

ADD/INCREASE

I love you even more because you may not always have felt wanted and loved at birth and always.

I love you even though your joy and purpose may seem hidden.

I love you even though you may not always have optimal energy level or body frequency.

I love you even though you may not always have optimal strength, connection, and compatibility with your True Self, Divine / Source, Spirit Guides, Angels, Nature Spirits, Animal Totems, and Magical Beings.

I love you even though you may sometimes have trouble with honesty and communication.

I love you even though you may not always have optimal compatibility of body cells and spin of the cells.

I love you even though you may not always have the optimal body and soul alignment with your original Blueprint.

I love you even though you may not always have optimal desire to live for the whole body, each organ, and each cell.

I love you even though you may not always have optimal connections with Positive Spirits such as Love, Freedom, Prosperity, Perfect Health, Peace, Joy, Harmony, Abundance, Passion, Romance, and Sex if age appropriate.

I love you even though you may not always have optimal positive patterns of attraction for things that help your highest good such as freedom, prosperity, optimal relationships including with your most compatible Soul Mate.

I love you even though you do not always peacefully and lovingly take care of yourself and your own needs and emotions first.

I love you even though you may not always have optimal amounts of beneficial bacteria.

I love you even though you may not always have optimal settings on all of your Allowing Meters.

I love you even though you may not always have optimal chemistry and communication throughout the entire body.

I love you even though you may not always have the optimal balance between the para-sympatric and sympatric nervous systems.

I love you even though you may not always have optimal absorption of the appropriate nutrients of all food and drink consumed to maintain ideal size and weight and chemistry.

I love you even though you may not always have the optimal knowledge, desire and ability to eat and drink only things that are good for you.

I love you even though you may not always have the ability to reprogram your body so that anything you do consume is right for you.

I love you even though you may not always have optimal levels of natural body lubrication.

I love you even though you may not always have optimal structural and spiritual alignment and the ability to autocorrect as needed.

I love you even though you may not always have the optimal ability to observe yourselves and knowledge, skill, and strength to make it right.

I love you even though you may not always remember your value does not decrease based on someone's inability to see your worth.

I love you even though you may not always remember that your words have power and ability to use them wisely. Therefore, eliminate bad and limiting self-talk and thought.

I love you even though you may not always have the optimal vision of time and space.

I love you even though you may not always have the optimal connection or recall of your higher purpose or the big picture.

I love you even though you may not always have the optimal knowledge, ability, and strength on how best to serve self, others, and the planet.

I love you even though you may not always have the optimal passion for life.

I love you even though you may not always have the optimal connection and knowledge for painless downloads.

I love you even though you may not always have optimal recall and execution of all Universal Laws and Symbols.

I love you even though you sometimes may forget the Law of Attraction and maybe really focusing on things you may not want.

I love you even though you may not always have optimal knowledge and execution of all Laws of Creation and any other Laws our higher self must follow.

I love you even though if you only focus on the problem, you might miss the easy solution.

I love you even though you may not always be able to automatically reset the body computer to ideal.

I love you even though you may not always have optimal faith.

I love you even though you may not always have optimal Love, courage, strength, knowledge, and wisdom in all things.

I love you even though you may struggle to allow joy and happiness into your life.

I love you even though you may not always remember and believe you deserve lightness, love, happiness, peace, harmony, and joy in your day to day life.

I love you even though you may not always make daily progress and development regarding your life purpose / dreams.

I love you even though you don't always attract what you expect, reflect what you desire, become what you respect, or mirror what you admire.

I love you even though you are not always surrounded with the dreamers and the doers, the thinks, but most of all, surround yourself with those who see the greatness within you, even when you don't see it yourself.

I love you even though not all your friends help you to find important things when you have lost them…. Your smile, your hope, and your courage.

I love you even though you may have forgotten passion isn't about finding the purpose for others in one's path, but letting your focus be on purpose and then passion will be found.

I love you even though you may have been under the illusion that "the truth that sets one free isn't the truth that other ones tells, but the truth that one confronts within yourself."

I love you even though you may not always be able to be in harmony with your spirit which is like a flowing river. You go where you will without pretense and arrives at your destination prepared to be yourself and only yourself. (Maya Angelou)

I love you even more because you may not always remember that your heart knows the way and you may not have the strength, knowledge, and ability to run in that direction. (Rumi)

I love you even though you may suffer from "PTSD - Post-Traumatic Sandy Disease."

OR THE SHORT FORM

I LOVE YOU EVEN MORE WHEN OTHERS MAY NOT ACCEPT LOVE IS YOUR RELIGION.
I LOVE YOU EVEN MORE WHEN YOU MAY NOT KNOW and REMEMBER IT.
I LOVE YOU EVEN WHEN YOU ARE NOT OVERFLOWING WITH SELF LOVE!!!
I LOVE YOU EVEN THOUGH YOU MAY BE AFRAID and PROGRAMMED NOT TO BE ABLE TO
- REMEMBER OR SEE YOUR TRUE SELF.
-EXPRESS YOUR LOVE TO OTHERS.
-BE ABLE TO LOVE YOURSELF.

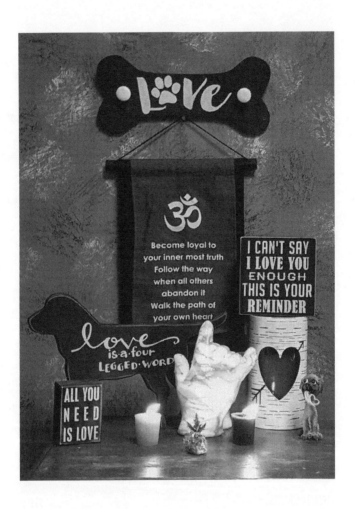

PROJECT # 4

SNELL BIBLICAL BASED LOVE FOR HEALING CHRISTIAN VERSION

Step 1 Clean the Soul.

I love you even though you, your loved ones and your lineage past present, and future may not always remember to use Jesus's Blood from the Cross to remove all Sins and all other things that do not serve your highest interest from your Souls. (Amen)

Step 2 Heal the Soul.

I love you even though you, your loved ones and your lineage past, present, and future may not always remember to use Jesus Resurrection Power of Dunamis to heal all wound of the Souls. (Amen)

Step 3 Clear the Area.

I love you even though you, your loved ones and your lineage past, present, and future may not always remember to ask God and all of His forms/helpers/ light beings to remove all of these things that no longer have anything in common with you. (Amen)

Step 4 Modified Archangel Michael Prayer.

I love you even though you, your loved ones and your lineage past, present, and future may not always remember to ask, Archangel Michael defend us in battle, be our protection from wickedness and snares of the Devil, cast into Hell Satan and all evil spirits including Agag, Balak, and Leviathan and all they are in contract with who rome throughout this world seeking the ruin of Souls. Amen.

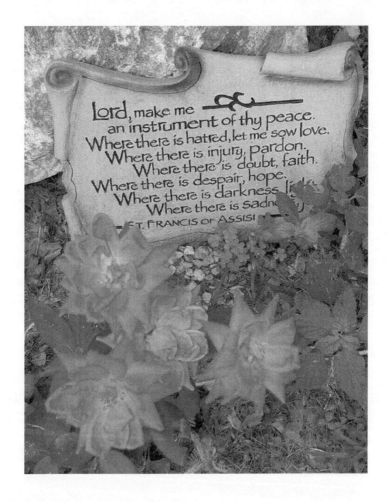

PROJECT # 5

SNELL BIBLICAL BASED LOVE FOR HEALING NEW AGE VERSION

Step 1 Clean the Soul.

I love you even though you, your loved ones, the lineage in every direction and all the possible incarnations thereof in all dimensions, time, space, and reality may not always remember to use Jesus's Blood from the Cross to remove all Sins and all other things that do not serve their highest interest from their Souls. (Amen)

Step 2 Heal the Soul.

I love you even though you, your loved ones, the lineage in every direction and all the possible incarnations thereof in all dimensions, time, space, and reality may not always remember to use Jesus Resurrection Power of Dunamis to heal all wound of the Souls. (Amen)

Step 3 Clear the Area.

I love you even though you, your loved ones, the lineage in every direction and all the possible incarnations thereof in all dimensions, time, space, and reality may not always remember to ask God and all of His forms/helpers/ light beings to remove all of these things that no longer have anything in common with you. (Amen)

Step 4 Modified Archangel Michael Prayer.

I love you even though you, your loved ones, the lineage in every direction and all the possible incarnations thereof in all dimensions, time, space, and reality may not always remember to ask, Archangel

Michael defend us in battle, be our protection from wickedness and snares of the Devil, cast into Hell Satan and all evil spirits including Agag, Balak, and Leviathan and all they are in contract with who rome throughout this world seeking the ruin of Souls. Amen.

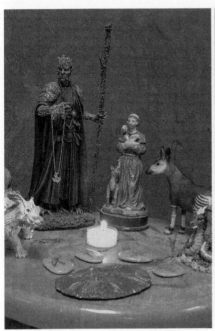
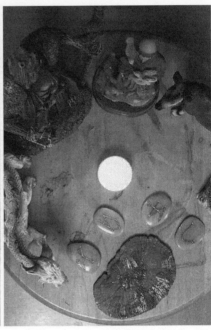

CLEAR HOME, CLEAR HEART, Learn to Clear the Energy of People and Places by Jean Haner

I first found out about Jean Haner during a Hay House World Summit 2017. I enjoyed listening to her, as I did almost all the other speakers I managed to hear. What made me buy her book was that she covered 5 Element / Traditional Chinese Medicine (TCM) for the soul. I was self-taught and then later became Certified in Veterinary Acupuncture. I am often amazed by how well it works, but was never taught or even thought about using it for the soul. Maybe because I learned Veterinary TCM the soul was not covered, even though I know animals have souls.

When the book arrived, its energy was so incredible. But no time to read it, so I tucked it behind the driver seat. Learning through osmosis is something I am always working on.

My daughter had multiple friends die in unrelated events within 48 hours of each other. I felt I just needed to take her away for the next weekend which happened to be an American holiday. So I took her to another country since we had passports and it won't be a holiday there. Throughout the entire extended weekend, a pattern was formed and repeated. It was so cool to be a part of and being able to notice it in real time was pure awesomeness. We would go someplace or do something. My daughter would get overwhelmed or tired. We would retreat to the hotel, where she would sleep, and I would read Clear Home, Clear Heart. I would be running my pendulum to clear all of us in the room while reading. I would finish a section, and my daughter would wake up. She would want to do exactly whatever it was I had just cleared. I made it through Part 1 Personal Clearing that weekend. After I came home, Spirit had me put together Cliff Notes for that section to understand where the problems might be. I did finish the book and recommended it to everyone. This book explains a lot of things in an easy to understand way.

Get JEAN HANER'S "CLEAR HOME, CLEAR HEART, Learn to clear the energy of people and Places" NOW.

PROJECT # 6

SNELL'S FIRST CLIFF NOTES
FOR JEAN HANER'S

"CLEAR HOME, CLEAR HEART, Learn to clear the energy of people and Places"

CLEAR 6 ENERGY FIELDS and 2 FINAL STEPS

1. <u>DISTURBING EFFECTS OF OTHERS</u>

2. <u>WATER</u>: *Fear, Trust, Ancestors, inherited Issues.*

3. <u>WOOD</u>: *Anger, Forgiveness, Vision* (hamster wheel).

4. <u>FIRE</u>: (Noise, crowds, and electric devices can affect your Fire energy.):

Love (Guardian of the Heart Gate),

Joy (Heart emotion) (slight imbalance: insomnia, anxiety or feeling of emotional instability; extremely imbalance: hysterical behavior, panic attacks, or post-traumatic stress disorder PTSD)

Healing the Heart (psychic like ability and shock absorber. imbalance: psychic boundaries altered. Psychic sponge, emotional overwhelmed, easily upset or scattered.)

5. <u>EARTH</u>: (Chinese Medicine Mother).

Safety (Imbalance: struggle with weight; accumulate home clutter; put thoughts into action or form lasting bonds.)

Support (imbalance could be lack of resources and a corresponding difficulty fulfilling your dreams, your lack of receptivity, you may exhaust yourself trying to do everything all by yourself.)

Relationships (may struggle with boundaries with others and feel guilty about tending to your own needs, you may over give, let people take advantage of you, or have trouble saying "no", worrying about others too much could lead to lost of your own strong center, may feel isolated and lonely without enough of a sense of connection to community. It is your mother who first teaches you the language of relationships, of how to give and receive in healthy ways.)

6. <u>METAL</u>: (Chinese Medicine for Father, or "Heaven or Sky")

Life Purpose (Each of us need to recognize that our so-called problems are the stepping stones that are showing the way and helping us evolve so we can fulfill our true calling. Imbalance: judgment, beliefs, critical inner voice, patterns of perfectionism or self – criticism, low self-worth.)

Authenticity (Feeling free to live your truth or feel a sense of the sacred in your life. Imbalance: thin skin, energy sensitive, frequent overwhelm, physical discomfort, allergies, environmental sensitivities, anxiety, hermit, standoffish, too controlling, needing everything your way.)

Recovering from Loss (Chinese Medicine emotion "grief." Imbalance: rigid, distant with others, cut off from your joy.)

7. <u>INTEGRATION</u> (The person's energy has been moving, shifting, releasing, and processing. It's important to create an opportunity for the changes to integrate within their system on every level.)

8. <u>GROUNDING</u> (Ground the person to make sure you leave them feeling complete and centered in their body and spirit.)

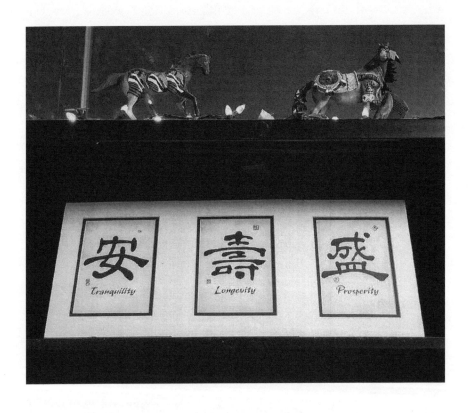

PROJECT # 7

SNELL'S SECOND CLIFF NOTES FOR JEAN HANER'S

"CLEAR HOME, CLEAR HEART, Learn to Clear the Energy of People And Places"

CLEAR 6 ENERGY FIELDS and 2 FINAL STEPS

1. <u>DISTURBING EFFECTS OF OTHERS</u>

2. <u>WATER</u>: *Fear, Trust, Ancestors, Inherited Issues.*

3. <u>WOOD</u>: *Anger, Forgiveness, Vision* (hamster wheel).

4. <u>FIRE</u>: (Noise, crowds, and electric devices can affect your Fire energy.)

Love (Guardian of the Heart Gate),

Joy (Imbalance: insomnia, anxiety or feeling of emotional instability, hysterical behavior, panic attacks, or post-traumatic stress disorder PTSD),

Healing the Heart (Imbalance: weakened psychic boundaries, psychic sponge, emotional overwhelmed, easily upset or scattered without knowing why.)

5. <u>EARTH</u>: (Mother).

Safety (Imbalance: weight, clutter, thoughts into action or form lasting bonds.)

Support (Imbalance: lack of resources and a corresponding difficulty fulfilling your dreams, your lack of receptivity, you may exhaust yourself trying to do everything all by yourself.)

Relationships (Imbalance: boundaries, guilty about tending to your own needs, over give, let people take advantage of you, trouble saying "no," worrying, lost of your strong center, isolated and lonely.)

6. <u>METAL</u>: (Father, or "Heaven or Sky").

Life Purpose (Imbalance was causing blocks with any issues that are preventing you from moving toward your life purpose: judgment, beliefs, critical inner voice, patterns of perfectionism or self – criticism, low self-worth.)

Authenticity (Imbalance: thin skin, energy sensitive, frequent overwhelm, physical discomfort, allergies, environmental sensitivities, anxiety, hermit, standoffish, too controlling, needing everything your way.)

Recovering from Loss (Imbalance: rigid, distant with others, cut off from your joy.)

7. <u>INTEGRATION</u>

8. <u>GROUNDING</u>

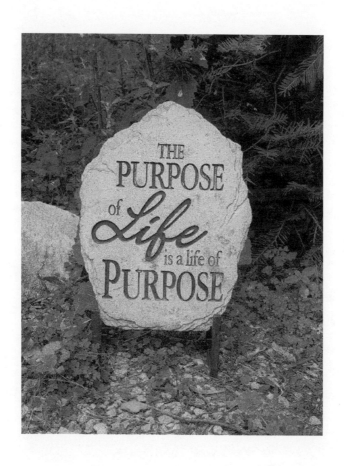

PROJECT # 8

DR. SNELL'S INSPIRED COMBINATION 10/12/2017

HO'OPONOPONO SIMPLE STATEMENT: I Love You. I am Sorry. Please forgive me. Thank you.
DR. SANDRA SNELL'S HO'OPONOPONO EXPANDED STATEMENT: I am That, I am. (or, I am _____, I am.) I Love You. I am Sorry. Please Forgive Me. Thank You. I release everything but the lessons and the LOVE. I Believe in Miracles. I Believe in You. I Believe in Me.

Step 1 Clean the Soul.

I am DISTURBING EFFECTS OF OTHERS, I am. I Love You. I am Sorry. Please Forgive Me. Thank You. I release everything but the lessons and the LOVE. I Believe in Miracles. I Believe in You. I Believe in Me.

I am WATER including Fear, Trust, Ancestors, and Inherited Issues, I am. I Love You. I am Sorry. Please Forgive Me. Thank You. I release everything but the lessons and the LOVE. I Believe in Miracles. I Believe in You. I Believe in Me.

I am WOOD including Anger, Forgiveness, and Vision, I am. I Love You. I am Sorry. Please Forgive Me. Thank You. I release everything but the lessons and the LOVE. I Believe in Miracles. I Believe in You. I Believe in Me.

I am FIRE including Love, Joy, and Heart Healing, I am. I Love You. I am Sorry. Please Forgive Me. Thank You. I release everything but the lessons and the LOVE. I Believe in Miracles. I Believe in You. I Believe in Me.

I am EARTH including Safety, Support, and Relationship, I am. I Love You. I am Sorry. Please Forgive Me. Thank You. I release everything but the lessons and the LOVE. I Believe in Miracles. I Believe in You. I Believe in Me.

I am METAL including Life Purpose, Authenticity, Grief, and Recovering from Loss, I am. I Love You. I am Sorry. Please Forgive Me. Thank You. I release everything but the lessons and the LOVE. I Believe in Miracles. I Believe in You. I Believe in Me.

I am Jesus' Blood from the Cross, I am. I Love You. I am Sorry. Please Forgive Me. Thank You. I release everything but the lessons and the LOVE. I Believe in Miracles. I Believe in You. I Believe in Me.

Step 2 Heal the Soul.

I am INTEGRATION, Balance and rebooting to perfect state, I am. I Love You. I am Sorry. Please Forgive Me. Thank You. I release everything but the lessons and the LOVE. I Believe in Miracles. I Believe in You. I Believe in Me.

I am Grounded, Complete, Centered, and fully connected to Source I am. I Love You. I am Sorry. Please Forgive Me. Thank You. I release everything but the lessons and the LOVE. I Believe in Miracles. I Believe in You. I Believe in Me.

I am Jesus' Resurrection Power of Dunamis, I am. I Love You. I am Sorry. Please Forgive Me. Thank You. I release everything but the lessons and the LOVE. I Believe in Miracles. I Believe in You. I Believe in Me.

Step 3 Strengthen the Light and Love Within.

I am SOURCE / GOD / CREATOR / DEVINE and all of its forms / helpers / Angels / light beings because they dwell inside me, I am. I Love You. I am Sorry. Please Forgive Me. Thank You. I release everything but the lessons and the LOVE. I Believe in Miracles. I Believe in You. I Believe in Me.

I am LOVE, LOVEABLE, LOVING, LOVELY, LOVED and a LOVER, I am. I Love You. I am Sorry. Please Forgive Me. Thank You. I release everything but the lessons and the LOVE. I Believe in Miracles. I Believe in You. I Believe in Me.

Step 4 Clear the Area and Modified Archangel Michael Prayer.

I ask SOURCE / God and all of His forms / helpers / light beings to remove all of these things that no longer have anything in common with me. (Amen)

Archangel Michael defend us in battle, be our protection from wickedness and snares of the Devil, cast into Hell Satan and all evil spirits including Agag, King Balak, and Leviathan and all they are in contract with, who rome throughout this world seeking the ruin of Souls. Amen.

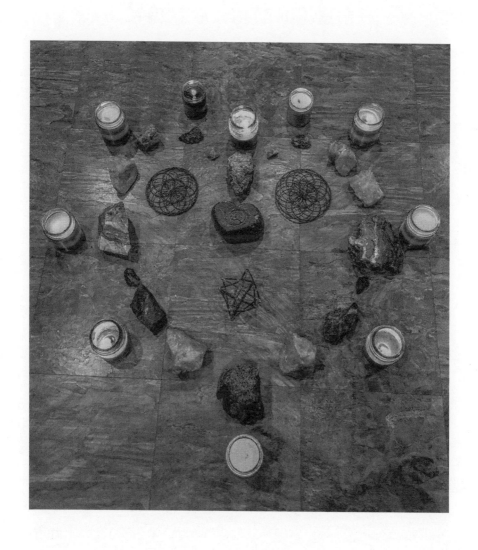

PROJECT # 9

DR. SNELL'S INSPIRED COMBINATION 4/1/2018

(Project # 8 with God Blessing)

HO'OPONOPONO SIMPLE STATEMENT: I Love You. I am Sorry. Please forgive me. Thank you.

DR. SANDRA SNELL'S HO'OPONOPONO EXPANDED STATEMENT on 4/1/2018: I am That, I am. (or, I am _____, I am.) I Love You. I am Sorry. Please Forgive Me. Thank You. I release everything but the lessons and the LOVE. I Believe in Miracles. I Believe in You. I Believe in Me. God Bless You and Me.

Step 1 Clean the Soul.

I am DISTURBING EFFECTS OF OTHERS, I am. I Love You. I am Sorry. Please Forgive Me. Thank You. I release everything but the lessons and the LOVE. I Believe in Miracles. I Believe in You. I Believe in Me. God Bless You and Me.

I am WATER including Fear, Trust, Ancestors, and Inherited Issues, I am. I Love You. I am Sorry. Please Forgive Me. Thank You. I release everything but the lessons and the LOVE. I Believe in Miracles. I Believe in You. I Believe in Me. God Bless You and Me.

I am WOOD including Anger, Forgiveness, and Vision, I am. I Love You. I am Sorry. Please Forgive Me. Thank You. I release everything but the lessons and the LOVE. I Believe in Miracles. I Believe in You. I Believe in Me. God Bless You and Me.

I am FIRE including Love, Joy, and Heart Healing, I am. I Love You. I am Sorry. Please Forgive Me. Thank You. I release everything but the lessons and the LOVE. I Believe in Miracles. I Believe in You. I Believe in Me. God Bless You and Me.

I am EARTH including Safety, Support, and Relationship, I am. I Love You. I am Sorry. Please Forgive Me. Thank You. I release everything but the lessons and the LOVE. I Believe in Miracles. I Believe in You. I Believe in Me. God Bless You and Me.

I am METAL including Life Purpose, Authenticity, Grief, and Recovering from Loss, I am. I Love You. I am Sorry. Please Forgive Me. Thank You. I release everything but the lessons and the LOVE. I Believe in Miracles. I Believe in You. I Believe in Me. God Bless You and Me.

I am Jesus' Blood from the Cross, I am. I Love You. I am Sorry. Please Forgive Me. Thank You. I release everything but the lessons and the LOVE. I Believe in Miracles. I Believe in You. I Believe in Me. God Bless You and Me.

Step 2 Heal the Soul.

I am INTEGRATION, Balance and rebooting to perfect state, I am. I Love You. I am Sorry. Please Forgive Me. Thank You. I release everything but the lessons and the LOVE. I Believe in Miracles. I Believe in You. I Believe in Me. God Bless You and Me.

I am Grounded, Complete, Centered, and fully connected to Source I am. I Love You. I am Sorry. Please Forgive Me. Thank You. I release everything but the lessons and the LOVE. I Believe in Miracles. I Believe in You. I Believe in Me. God Bless You and Me.

I am Jesus' Resurrection Power of Dunamis, I am. I Love You. I am Sorry. Please Forgive Me. Thank You. I release everything but the lessons and the LOVE. I Believe in Miracles. I Believe in You. I Believe in Me. God Bless You and Me.

Step 3 Strengthen the Light and Love Within.

I am SOURCE / GOD / CREATOR / DEVINE and all of its forms / helpers / Angels / light beings because they dwell inside me, I am. I Love You. I am Sorry. Please Forgive Me. Thank You. I release everything but the lessons and the LOVE. I Believe in Miracles. I Believe in You. I Believe in Me. God Bless You and Me.

I am LOVE, LOVEABLE, LOVING, LOVELY, LOVED and a LOVER, I am. I Love You. I am Sorry. Please Forgive Me. Thank You. I release everything but the lessons and the LOVE. I Believe in Miracles. I Believe in You. I Believe in Me. God Bless You and Me.

Step 4 Clear the Area and Modified Archangel Michael Prayer.

I ask SOURCE / God and all of His forms / helpers / light beings to remove all of these things that no longer have anything in common with me. (Amen)

Archangel Michael defend us in battle, be our protection from wickedness and snares of the Devil, cast into Hell Satan and all evil spirits including Agag, King Balak, and Leviathan and all they are in contract with, who rome throughout this world seeking the ruin of Souls. Amen.

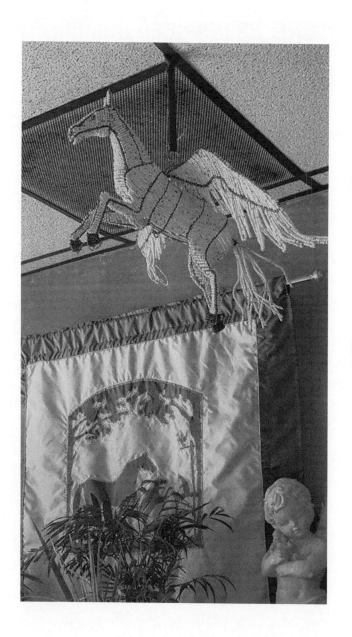

PROJECT # 10

DR. SNELL'S INSPIRED COMBINATION
4/19/2018 & 7/25/2018

HO'OPONOPONO SIMPLE STATEMENT: I Love You. I am Sorry. Please forgive me. Thank you.

DR. SANDRA SNELL'S HO'OPONOPONO EXPANDED STATEMENT: I am That, I am. (or, I am _____, I am.) I Love You. I am Sorry. Please Forgive Me. Thank You. I am Worthy. I release everything but the lessons and the LOVE. I Believe in Miracles. I Believe in You. I Believe in Me. I am Enough. God Bless You and Me.

Step 1 Clean Body (Face the "Dragons" and feed them to let them free)

I am all things in the body, I am. I Love You. I am Sorry. Please Forgive Me. Thank You. I am Worthy. I release everything but the lessons and the LOVE. I Believe in Miracles. I Believe in You. I Believe in Me. I am Enough. God Bless You and Me.

I am all SEVEN KARMIC SHADOWS: Abuse; Addiction; Violence; Poverty; Illness; Abandonment; Betrayal, I am. I Love You. I am Sorry. Please Forgive Me. Thank You. I am Worthy. I release everything but the lessons and the LOVE. I Believe in Miracles. I Believe in You. I Believe in Me. I am Enough. God Bless You and Me. (You may want to repeat for each individual Karmic Shadow and possibly repeat the troubled ones as needed.) (Sara Wiseman)

I am all emotions, I am. I Love You. I am Sorry. Please Forgive Me. Thank You. I am Worthy. I release everything but the lessons and the LOVE. I Believe in Miracles. I Believe in You. I Believe in Me. I am

Enough. God Bless You and Me. (You may want to include the problem emotions.)

I am all fears, I am. I Love You. I am Sorry. Please Forgive Me. Thank You. I am Worthy. I release everything but the lessons and the LOVE. I Believe in Miracles. I Believe in You. I Believe in Me. I am Enough. God Bless You and Me. (You may want to include the problem fears.)

I am all doubts, I am. I Love You. I am Sorry. Please Forgive Me. Thank You. I am Worthy. I release everything but the lessons and the LOVE. I Believe in Miracles. I Believe in You. I Believe in Me. I am Enough. God Bless You and Me. (You may want to include the problem doubts.)

I am all blocks, I am. I Love You. I am Sorry. Please Forgive Me. Thank You. I am Worthy. I release everything but the lessons and the LOVE. I Believe in Miracles. I Believe in You. I Believe in Me. I am Enough. God Bless You and Me. (You may want to include the problem blocks.)

I am hopelessness, I am. I Love You. I am Sorry. Please Forgive Me. Thank You. I am Worthy. I release everything but the lessons and the LOVE. I Believe in Miracles. I Believe in You. I Believe in Me. I am Enough. God Bless You and Me.

I am helplessness, I am. I Love You. I am Sorry. Please Forgive Me. Thank You. I am Worthy. I release everything but the lessons and the LOVE. I Believe in Miracles. I Believe in You. I Believe in Me. I am Enough. God Bless You and Me.

I am worthlessness, I am. I Love You. I am Sorry. Please Forgive Me. Thank You. I am Worthy. I release everything but the lessons and the LOVE. I Believe in Miracles. I Believe in You. I Believe in Me. I am Enough. God Bless You and Me.

I am all possible diseases, sensitivities, and allergies, I am. I Love You. I am Sorry. Please Forgive Me. Thank You. I am Worthy. I release everything but the lessons and the LOVE. I Believe in Miracles. I

Believe in You. I Believe in Me. I am Enough. God Bless You and Me. (You may want to include individual problems.)

I am free of all things that do not serve my highest good, I am. I Love You. I am Sorry. Please Forgive Me. Thank You. I am Worthy. I release everything but the lessons and the LOVE. I Believe in Miracles. I Believe in You. I Believe in Me. I am Enough. God Bless You and Me.

Step 2 Heal the Body

I am a perfect Child of Source / Divine / God, I am. I Love You. I am Sorry. Please Forgive Me. Thank You. I am Worthy. I release everything but the lessons and the LOVE. I Believe in Miracles. I Believe in You. I Believe in Me. I am Enough. God Bless You and Me.

I am a living temple for Source / Divine / God to dwell, I am. I Love You. I am Sorry. Please Forgive Me. Thank You. I am Worthy. I release everything but the lessons and the LOVE. I Believe in Miracles. I Believe in You. I Believe in Me. I am Enough. God Bless You and Me.

I am fully connected to all of my perfectly functioning chakras and DNA, I am. I Love You. I am Sorry. Please Forgive Me. Thank You. I am Worthy. I release everything but the lessons and the LOVE. I Believe in Miracles. I Believe in You. I Believe in Me. I am Enough. God Bless You and Me.

I am constantly receiving and utilizing everything my body requires for optimal health, even if just energetically, I am. I Love You. I am Sorry. Please Forgive Me. Thank You. I am Worthy. I release everything but the lessons and the LOVE. I Believe in Miracles. I Believe in You. I Believe in Me. I am Enough. God Bless You and Me.

I am Enough, I am. I Love You. I am Sorry. Please Forgive Me. Thank You. I am Worthy. I release everything but the lessons and the LOVE. I Believe in Miracles. I Believe in You. I Believe in Me. I am Enough. God Bless You and Me.

I am Worthy, I am. I Love You. I am Sorry. Please Forgive Me. Thank You. I am Worthy. I release everything but the lessons and the LOVE. I Believe in Miracles. I Believe in You. I Believe in Me. I am Enough. God Bless You and Me.

I am beautiful, fit and healthy, I am. I Love You. I am Sorry. Please Forgive Me. Thank You. I am Worthy. I release everything but the lessons and the LOVE. I Believe in Miracles. I Believe in You. I Believe in Me. I am Enough. God Bless You and Me.

I am Peace, Love, and Joy, I am. I Love You. I am Sorry. Please Forgive Me. Thank You. I am Worthy. I release everything but the lessons and the LOVE. I Believe in Miracles. I Believe in You. I Believe in Me. I am Enough. God Bless You and Me.

Step 3 Clean the Soul.

I am DISTURBING EFFECTS OF OTHERS, I am. I Love You. I am Sorry. Please Forgive Me. Thank You. I am Worthy. I release everything but the lessons and the LOVE. I Believe in Miracles. I Believe in You. I Believe in Me. I am Enough. God Bless You and Me.

I am WATER including Fear, Trust, Ancestors, and Inherited Issues, I am. I Love You. I am Sorry. Please Forgive Me. Thank You. I am Worthy. I release everything but the lessons and the LOVE. I Believe in Miracles. I Believe in You. I Believe in Me. I am Enough. God Bless You and Me.

I am WOOD including Anger, Forgiveness, and Vision, I am. I Love You. I am Sorry. Please Forgive Me. Thank You. I am Worthy. I release everything but the lessons and the LOVE. I Believe in Miracles. I Believe in You. I Believe in Me. I am Enough. God Bless You and Me.

I am FIRE including Love, Joy, and Heart Healing, I am. I Love You. I am Sorry. Please Forgive Me. Thank You. I am Worthy. I release everything but the lessons and the LOVE. I Believe in Miracles. I Believe in You. I Believe in Me. I am Enough. God Bless You and Me.

I am EARTH including Safety, Support, and Relationship, I am. I Love You. I am Sorry. Please Forgive Me. Thank You. I am Worthy. I release everything but the lessons and the LOVE. I Believe in Miracles. I Believe in You. I Believe in Me. I am Enough. God Bless You and Me.

I am METAL including Life Purpose, Authenticity, Grief, and Recovering from Loss, I am. I Love You. I am Sorry. Please Forgive Me. Thank You. I am Worthy. I release everything but the lessons and the LOVE. I Believe in Miracles. I Believe in You. I Believe in Me. I am Enough. God Bless You and Me.

I am Jesus' Blood from the Cross, I am. I Love You. I am Sorry. Please Forgive Me. Thank You. I am Worthy. I release everything but the lessons and the LOVE. I Believe in Miracles. I Believe in You. I Believe in Me. I am Enough. God Bless You and Me.

Step 4 Heal the Soul.

I am INTEGRATION, Balance and Rebooting to perfect state, I am. I Love You. I am Sorry. Please Forgive Me. Thank You. I am Worthy. I release everything but the lessons and the LOVE. I Believe in Miracles. I Believe in You. I Believe in Me. I am Enough. God Bless You and Me.

I am Grounded, Complete, Centered, and fully connected to Source I am. I Love You. I am Sorry. Please Forgive Me. Thank You. I am Worthy. I release everything but the lessons and the LOVE. I Believe in Miracles. I Believe in You. I Believe in Me. I am Enough. God Bless You and Me.

I am Jesus' Resurrection Power of Dunamis, I am. I Love You. I am Sorry. Please Forgive Me. Thank You. I am Worthy. I release everything but the lessons and the LOVE. I Believe in Miracles. I Believe in You. I Believe in Me. I am Enough. God Bless You and Me.

Step 5 Strengthen the Light and Love Within.

I am SOURCE / GOD / CREATOR / DEVINE and all of its forms / helpers / Angels / light beings because they dwell inside me, I am. I Love You. I am Sorry. Please Forgive Me. Thank You. I am Worthy. I release everything but the lessons and the LOVE. I Believe in Miracles. I Believe in You. I Believe in Me. I am Enough. God Bless You and Me.

I am LOVE, LOVEABLE, LOVING, LOVELY, LOVED and a LOVER, I am. I Love You. I am Sorry. Please Forgive Me. Thank You. I am Worthy. I release everything but the lessons and the LOVE. I Believe in Miracles. I Believe in You. I Believe in Me. I am Enough. God Bless You and Me.

Step 6 Clear the Area and Modified Archangel Michael Prayer.

I ask God and all of His forms / helpers / light beings to remove all of these things that no longer have anything in common with me. (Amen).

Archangel Michael defend us in battle, be our protection from wickedness and snares of the Devil, cast into Hell Satan and all evil spirits including Agag, King Balak, and Leviathan and all they are in contract with, who rome throughout this world seeking the ruin of Souls. Amen.

Now that I am free of all beliefs, Identifications, and Attachments to things that do not serve my highest good. I hereby activate and awaken all 108 Chakras and crystalline DNA, fully grounded into the pure crystalline core of the 5th dimensional Earth plane, where I step forward as a light bearer of Light Center Consciousness. Calling forth my most life fulfilling reality, for the wellbeing of all. That I am now. And so it is…. (Matt Kahn).

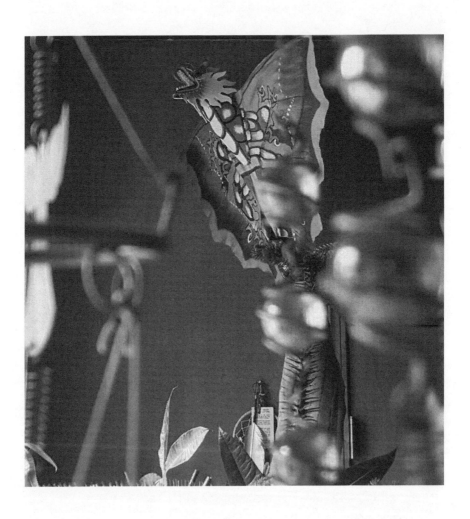

PROJECT # 11

DR. SNELL'S DOWSING
HEALING GUIDE 2/2018

The initial intent is to direct this energy to _____, their family, animals, home, property, work, and projects in all time, space, realities, and dimensions...

Permission is asked for this to be done. If denied, by intended receiver, Permission is asked again to their "Higher Selves". If denied again, continue for yourself. The only one you can truly change is yourself. However, since we are all One, by changing yourself, hopefully the intended receiver will also benefit..... Or by looking at it from Ho'oponopono theory, you take full responsibility for everything and everyone, so working on yourself, will help others...

All bodies including physical, mental, emotional, spiritual, light, sound bodies and all others known and not known are to be address.
Activate and awaken all 108 Chakras and crystalline DNA, yet stay fully grounded. (Matt Kahn)
Increase the ability to connect with Universal Chakras and all others known and unknown.
Activate all available energies, forces, systems, programs, areas, regions, meridians and points known and unknown that would be beneficial to healing.(ie. MAP: The Co-Creative White Brotherhood Medical Assistance Program, Access Bars, Reiki, Chinese Medicine, Ayurvedic Medicine, Tapping, T Touch, etc.)
Increase ability to remember that "everyone is perfect. What is not perfect is the data or memory." (Ho'oponopono)
Increase ability to love, apologize, forgive, appreciate, accept, bless and be grateful to self, others, and devine. (Ho'oponopono)

Remove negative entities, negative forces, poltergeist, Demonic Kings, attachments, beacons, toxic chords, implants, non beneficial E. T. s and either revert them back to 100% prue light or deal with them as needed to no longer be able to harm others.

Bring soul to this dimension. Fix fragmentations of soul. Return missing Soul pieces. Remove all Sins from the Soul. Heal all wounds of the Soul. Soul becomes whole, healed, complete, grounded, perfect, strong, Dunamis, and compatible with body and self.

Increase ability to remember to Ask for Source / Divine / ArchAngels / Angels / Spirit Guides / Ascended Masters / White Light works assistance. Because of Free Will, if they are not asked, they can not help. Strengthen the Light and Love Within SOURCE / GOD / CREATOR / DIVINE and all of its forms / helpers / Angels / light beings / Ascended Masters / etc.

Increase ability to remember everyone, including self is LOVE, LOVEABLE, LOVING, LOVELY, LOVED and a LOVER.

Increase receiver's desire for improvement and decrease their resistance to your help.

Adjust surface tension of water to eliminate non beneficial memory of water in body of trauma of this life and past lives. (negative cellular memory)

Activate the genes that need to activated. Deactivate the genes that need to be deactivated.

Increase ability to learn from life lessons when delivered at a whisper, instead of waiting for the two by four or steam roller.

Increase ability to remember that everything is place in front of us to learn and grow.

Increase ability to "Love whatever Arises." (Matt Kahn)

Increase ability to release everything but the lessons and the Love. (Doreen Virtue)

Increase ability to remember not to take personal what is being yelled at you, because they are just telling you what they need deep down to heal. (Matt Kahn)

Reprogram body to create an energy field around it that transforms all non-beneficial energy sent to it or already within it into the most appropriate energy needed at the time.

Reprogram body to automatically reset all Allowing Meters to current ideal settings.

Reprogram body to automatically re-establish to every molecule within it the statement, "I am Love, Joyful, Beautiful, Healthy, Worthy, Intelligent, and Enough!!!!."""

FORGIVE / TRANSMUTE / RELEASE / REMOVE / REDUCE / NEUTRALIZE NON BENEFICIAL EFFECTS

Negative energetic patterns, negative patterns of attraction, and negative thought forms, negative Imprints, Intrusions.

Curses, hexes, spells, black magic, witchcraft, bad medicine, attachments, hooks, daggers.

Negative Vortexes, Geopathic Stress, Negative Hartman & Curry Lines, Negative Interference Line, Negative Energy Forms in properties. (Marie Diamond)

Battle Energies held by nature and body, released with gentleness and ease.

Karmic Shadows: Abuse; Addiction; Violence; Poverty; Illness; Abandonment; Betrayal. (Sara Wiseman)

Disturbing effects of others.

Stress of all kinds including geographic (water veins), Electromagnetic, A. C. current, sonar, Non beneficial Spirit Guides, archetypes, psychic chords/ toxic chords, programming / brainwashing, Negative karmic influences, Old vows or agreements including poverty, chastity, obedience, loyalty, suffering, etc.

Effect of heritage, culture, & religion of ancestors and self.

Belief, thought, & memories including inherited, self imposed, or by association.

All forms of repression and imprisonment including self imposed.

Self-sabotage, self-destruct, self-hate, & self punishment mental programs.

Spirits of victimization, co-dependency, disease, and emotions such as anger, greed, grief, unworthiness, doubt, shame, guilt, and fear including fear of success and fear of failure.

Miasmas, disease processes, addictions, excess body fat, non beneficial bacteria, viruses (Epstein Barr and all of its forms known and unknown, Lymes, Herpes, Poxs, Papilloma, HIV, influenza, Inherited viruses etc.).

Fungus, parasites, diabetes, allergies, sensitivities.

Adrenal Fatigue.

Meningeal Adhesions, trigger points, blocked energy flow, blocked mardians.

All chemical, biological, & radiological pollutants of water / body.

Non beneficial effects of vaccines, dental work, medications, supplements, herbs, oils, etc.

Toxins in Your Body: heavy metals; persistent organic pollutants; opertoninic organisms (bacteria, yeast, fungus, mycoplasma, candida); energetic toxins; emotional / spiritual toxins; food toxins; environmental toxins, inherited toxins.

Epstein Barr Virus and all of its cofactors including Cytomegalovirus, H. pylori, Strep B bacteria, candida, mercury toxicity, cadmium toxicity, lead toxicity, aluminum toxicity, copper toxicity and possible allergies to each.

Food causing Toxicity; GMO, Hybridized and processed grains; alcohol; all processed foods and drinks; low quality supplements; artificial sweeteners; conventional animal products; all refined sugars; refined processed oils; low quality protein products.

Catarrhal Mucoid Plaque and all other places where negative emotions maybe trapped in the body. (Green Smoothie Girl, Robyn Openshaw)

All blocks to unlimited abundance including, but not limited too: Resistance; Doubt and Fear;' Fear of Change; Money Zapping Decisions; Fear of Growth; Fear of Success; Fear of Rejection; Fear of Numbers; Indecision; Feeling Stuck; unclear Values; unclear Future; Clutter; Family Blocks; Blame; unknowing the Ultimate You; unclear Future Self; Turning Blocks into Profits; Self Sabotage; Lack of Self Worth; Financial Mess; Financial Illusions; Fear of Scarcity; Welcoming Abundance. (Christie Marie Sheldon)

The 4 Traps of Self-Doubt: Hesitating; Hiding; Hypercritical; Helplessness. (Mel Robbins)

The Top 10 Self-Limiting Beliefs: I'm too old; I'm not smart enough; I'm not educated enough; I'm afraid of trying and failing; You have to have money to make money; I've already tried everything; It's selfish of me to want more; I don't feel that I really deserve it; I don't have the willpower; All the good ones are taken. (Mary Morrissey)

C - reactive protein, Inflammation.

Autoimmune Antibodies and /or the non beneficial effect of Antibodies that made cross react to self or needed proteins for healthy bodies.

Hertz frequency effect on people and animals.

BALANCE / IDEAL LEVEL:

Universal energy - polarity, aura / clear holes, pH, body chemistry, metabolism.

Mind, body, and Soul via Traditional Chinese Medicine, 5 Element, and any other treatment system know and unknown.

Life Structures: Spiritual, Ego, Livelihood, Relationship, Body Temple, Financial, Beliefs, Community, etc.

Body senses including hearing, vision, taste, touch, and smell.

Body systems including matrix, lymphatic, nervous, respiratory, digestive, endocrine, urological, circulatory, dermatological, hematological, etc.

Glands Including hypothalamus, pineal, thyroid, adrenal, reproductive, etc.

Hormones including serotonin, noradrenaline, melatonin, etc.

Brain chemistry, brain blood flow, and right and left hemispheres.

Neurotransmitters: Dopamine; Serotonin; Acetylcholine; GABA.

Command Center including messages from brain to body (stroke).

Red and white blood cells, lithium, and amino acids.

Chakras, assemblage point, hara line, electrons.

Angiogenesis (blood vessel growth) (Excessive leads to; cancer, blinging diseases, psoriasis, arthritis, endometriosis, AIDS- Kaposi sarcoma, Alzheimer's Disease, obesity, multiple sclerosis, cerebral malais, rossesa) (Insufficient leads to; chronic wound, coronary heart disease, peripheral arterial disease, stroke, neuropathies, preeclampsia, hair loss, erectile dysfunction).

Microbiome.

Permeability of Gut membrane and Blood Brain Barrier.
Body weight & size to ideal.
Sleep - quality and quantity.
Light body & Sound body.
Soil Balanced and Stabilized.

ADD / INCREASE / IMPROVE / GROW / EXPAND

Energy level.
Spontaneous Remission and / or Spontaneous Healing.
Body Frequency.
Oxygen to the cells as if in Hyperbaric or Ozone therapy.
Natural Killer Cells.
Natural continuous Infusion of Stem Cells.
Strength of Nature Spirits, Guides, Angels, Magical Beings.
Compatibility and Communication with all beneficial guides (yours and others).
Connection with Source / Divine / true higher self / Mother Earth.
Ability to easily and swiftly move to higher Levels of Consciousness, from Victim to Manifestation, from Manifestation to Channeling, and from Channeling to Being. (Michael Beckwith)
Degree of feeling wanted at birth and always.
Compatibility of body cells / spin of the cells, beneficial bacteria.
Implant & Activate cetyl - myristoleate (a mouse fatty acid that prevents them from getting arthritis)
Your body's desire to live, whole, each organ, each cell, etc.
Beneficial effects of vaccines, dental work, medications, supplements, herbs, oils, etc.
Your body's alignment with your original blueprint.
Body's ability to stay in alignment and ability to fix itself as needed.
Our ability to observe ourselves and knowledge, ability, and strength to make it right.
Positive Spirits including love, freedom, prosperity, perfect health, peace, joy, harmony, abundance, romance, passion, and sex (if age appropriate), etc.
Desire and Ability to do and consume what is best for our body.

Ho'oponopono Cleaning Tools number, availability, strength, etc.

Ability to use all Universal Laws and Symbols known and unknown to our benefit, including the Law of One or Oneness, the Law of Radiance, the Law of Attraction, and the Law of Allowing, etc.

Ability to Live in the Moment and be Mindful.

The willingness and capability to do The Progress Principle – make progress on at least one thing that truly matters to you each day.

Serenity to accept the things that cannot change, Courage to change the things that can, and the Wisdom to know the difference.

Wisdom to know when if told it "cannot be changed" by another human or society, if it is really true or not.

Ability to remember Chinese proverb "The person who says it cannot be done, should not interrupt the person doing it."

Ability to remember "If you have a health concern, that the inner power that embryologically once built your body is the same power that can rebuild your body." (Dr. John Demartini)

Limitless ability to conquer challenges; and infinite potential to succeed.

Ability to remember, understand and execute: "When I run after what I think I want, my days are a furnace of distress and anxiety. If I sit in my own place of patience what I need flows to me, and without any pain. From this I understand what I want also wants me, is looking for me and attracting me. There is a Great Secret in this for anyone who can grasp it." (Rumi)

Bio availability of everything we consume to be the very best and what is needed; Organic, non- allergenic, sugar free, gluten free, litichen free, cruelty free animal products, Fair Trade, good Fats, MCT, Medicinal mushrooms (lion's mane chaga, etc), Vitamins, Minerals, quercetin, berberine, curcumin, resveratrol, iodine, low - dose lithium CFA, oligomeric procyanidins compounds, boswellia, niacin, Vit G, etc. and all others know and unknown.

Reprogram our body that everything we consume is good or neutral for us.

LAST STEPS

REBOOT THE BODY COMPUTER TO THE IDEAL SETTINGS!
Loop process as often as needed.

I am That, I am. I Love You. I am Sorry. Please Forgive Me. Thank You. I am Worthy. I release everything but the lessons and the LOVE. I Believe in Miracles. I Believe in You. I Believe in Me. I am Enough. God Bless You.

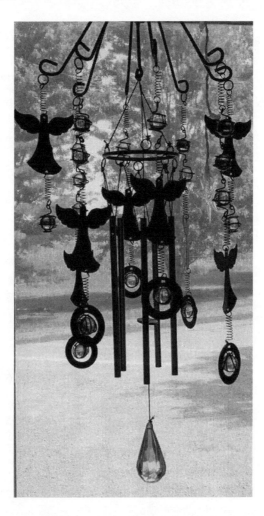

PROJECT # 12

DR. SNELL'S DOWSING OF LAND AND INHABITANTS

Make or get an aerial map of the property to be cleared. Google maps have made this easy.

For my own, I have also roughly drawn out each floor / level of the buildings showing the different rooms. (Not to scale).

Find an ample space to work; often it is not large enough. I use my Animal Hospital's exam table, with a handy healing vortex real close by.

Raise vibration by applying Essential Oils. I use doTERRA Immortelle, my Ho'oponopono Cleaning Oil Mixture, and any others Spirit wants.

Light at least one candle.

Spirit lead collecting of objects, tools, or whatever may be needed for this upcoming process.

Center and ground with pendulum in dominant hand. I often use my seven directions brief ceremony described in Tools, but repeated here.

""Spirit" (my Guides, Angels, Inner Voice, Creator, Source, etc.) has given me a Native American 7 direction very brief ceremony. Often this can be done in less than a minute. Sometimes I do not know what direction East is for my starting point. That is when I will close my eyes, spin slowly in a circle until I feel or hear stop for a good starting point.

Stand facing East / Where the Sun rises from, in a vortex or favorite spot if possible, but where ever will work. I place my hands outstretched palms up. I give love and great gratitude, during which I am pulled forward. I ask, often mentally, for all that is needed to walk in balance for this day, during which I am pushed backward. When I can stand straight, I turn right a quarter turn (90 degrees), repeat for South. Turn right a quarter turn, repeat for West / where the sun sets. Turn right a quarter turn, repeat for North. Aim hands, face and eyes to the ground, grow or reconnect the roots from your body into the center of Mother Earth. Release all things that no longer serve your highest good through those roots back into Mother Earth. Repeat the process of giving love, great gratitude and asking for balance. Aim hands, face and eyes to above, open up your crown chakra and reconnect with all great things above that dwells in Father Sky. Repeat the process. Put hands on the abdomen, repeat for the Great Mystery Within and the Body Temple where Source / Creator / God / Divine are invited to live. Take a moment to be in that space thoroughly Loved, Supported, Connected and in Balance."

There is a prayer I often used for my Group Healing Sessions, that could be useful here:

I give thanks to those that I am about to invite!
I ask that this room, this home, or building and the grounds become a sacred space.
I invite the Divine to be present.
I invite Great Spirit, Mother Father God to be present.
I invite Great Mystery to be present.
I invite the Compassionate and loving Ancestors to be present, and I give thanks to them because without them we couldn't be here.
I invite the Great Teachers and Master to be present, especially those that we have connections to and affiliations with.
I invite the Angels, the great beings of light, especially the Archangels, the Guardian Angels and the Angels of Healing.
I invite the Power Animals, the Totems, and I give thanks to them for loaning their power, their qualities, and for the relationship.
I invite the Healing Spirits of all the realms, and give thanks for the healing that I know is going to happen.
I invite the Elements: Earth, Water, Fire, Air, Metal, and Sacred Space. And I ask for a balancing of the Elements.
I invite the Compassionate Spirits and Devas.

I invite the Earth, the Sun, and the Moon.
I give thanks to the Stars and the Compassionate Star People.
I invite the Directions and the Guardians of the Directions.
I invite the Four Great Winds.
I give thanks to the Great Spirits of the Land, and I ask to be in harmony with you and to prosper here.
I give thanks to the Spirits of this place for allowing this work to happen here.
And as always, I give thanks in advance for the blessings that I know will happen here.
Thank you!
(Aho) (Amen) (Awomen)

Invite in your Higher Self.

Place the maps and drawings of your property in the center of the table with North facing North.

Invite in East, place paper and / or objects representing East on the East side of the table.
The directions can represent different things to different tribes, religions, beliefs, etc.
East on the paper I use has; Element - Air; Season - Spring; Herb - Tobacco; Animal - Eagle / Hawk; Tree - Yellow Birch; Crystal - Cat's Eye; Angel - Uriel; Clan - Butterfly. (Bluehawks Specs)

Invite in South, place paper and / or objects representing South on the South side of the table.
South: Element - Fire; Season - Summer; Herb - Sage; Animal - Wolf / Mouse; Tree - White Fir; Crystal - Geode; Angel - Raphael; Clan - Thunderbird. (Bluehawks Specs)

Invite in West, place paper and / or objects representing West on the West side of the table.
West: Element - Water; Season - Fall; Herb - Cedar; Animal - Bear / Thunder Beings; Tree - Black Willow; Crystal - Aquamarine; Angel - Gabriel; Clan - Frog. (Bluehawks Specs)

Invite in North, place paper and / or objects representing North on the North side of the table.

North: Element - Earth; Season - Winter; Herb - Sweetgrass; Animal - Buffalo; Tree - Red Oak; Crystal - Amethyst; Angel - Michael; Clan - Turtle. (Bluehawks Specs)

Invite in all else of 100% pure Light needed for this clearing including Higher Selves of all inhabitants.

Test the Energy level of whole and if want each part.

From here on I follow Spirit or Channel so order and everything can vary greatly.

However, basic things that need to be checked, adjusted to ideal by either clear, forgive, compassion, gratitude, love, transform, release or strengthening, and then balance to ideal would include: Demonic Kings, poltergeist, ghost, ley lines, EMT, negative vortexes, Geopathic stress, negative Hartman lines, negative curry lines, Interference lines, Battle energy, negative trapped energy, underground water, Energy flow blocks, Bloodstones, ley line intersections, non beneficial beacons, etc. I will start by doing this for the entire area. I may then hold the pendulum over the maps or drawings and ask if more is needed in a certain place and if so where and what. Do as your answers lead, making sure all answers are of the light.

Recheck Energy level as above.

Check if you should do any other of my projects. If yes, Figure out which one by asking which number with a dowsing chart or merely asking do I need to do project # 1 - 11 one at a time with yes / no. If yes, do that project.

Recheck Energy level as above.

Check if you should do any other of my projects. If yes, repeat as above. If no, continue to next step.

Recheck Energy level as above.

Check to see if there is anything that was missed that you can get the memo to fix now.

Recheck Energy level if anything else was done.

Ask if this could remain a Sacred Place. When a place becomes Sacred, you may feel different / more peace, you may smell a change in the air / like after rain, and you may hear an echo to tones or song.

If you are doing your property go to Final Steps.

If you are doing this for someone else's property make sure you have dowsed your own enough times there will not be any problems. If Cleared to go forward lay their maps and / or drawings on top of your cleaned maps and / or drawings.

Hold pendulum over a candle until clear or done moving.

Invite in all else of the Light needed for this clearing including Higher Selves of all inhabitants.

Go back to: Test the Energy level of whole and if want each part.

Final Steps

HA Breathing with all 6 finger connections.

Thank all that came to help in the process. Release them to go, but they are welcome to stay and return as often as they want.

Hold pendulum over a candle until clear or done moving.

I am That, I am. I Love You. I am Sorry. Please Forgive Me. Thank You. I am Worthy. I release everything but the lessons and the LOVE.

I Believe in Miracles. I Believe in You. I Believe in Me. I am Enough. God Bless You and Me.

And So It Is.

Aho.

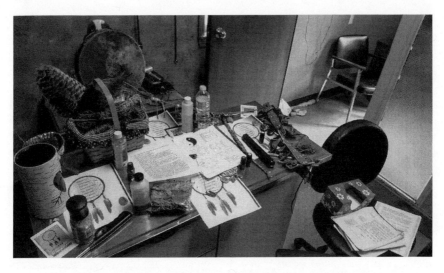

Picture after a Land Cleaning Ceremony 6/2017

Our Health Path Thus Far

Life is about the Journey. You can meet each new thing as an obstacle or a lesson. The thing does not change either way. The only part that changes is your opinion of it. During some of my daughters darkest days, people who knew and people who did not know would ask me, "How are you?" My response would be the same for either group asking the question. "I am trying to walk through my lessons with Love."

Being a Holistic Veterinarian, Reiki Master, Shaman practitioner and so much more, handing my daughter over to Western Medicine current Hospital Systems was heartbreaking. I was in sheer panic over my daughter's life and well being. But when I took time to breathe and look, there were so many signs, we were not alone. The Divine Timing of a Christmas gift I sent over a month late to a dear person, who opened the package, and sent me the most beautiful loving text just as I walked out of the Hospital the first time. It reminded me I was not alone, I was Loved, and reading it let me cry for the first time. My guides just kept repeating, "This is needed for growth, everything will be alright." Another time in the ER we were waiting for hours and hours. In about the middle of it, the clock above her head changed to a different time and stopped there for at least an hour. It was still stopped when I left to run home for things and a quick shower. During the shower it came to me, that was the time my daughter could have died if not for her Army of Angels. When I returned the clock was right on track again. I also sat in a different spot than earlier, where I saw massive energy waves only over my daughter. It looked like what I see when I look at silos. I grew up in Florida without silos, so I do not know if, I have seen this my whole life or not. I also never talked about this ability to others before this, because I just thought everyone saw this wavey stuff that hurts your eyes over silos.

Oh, believe me, I am human. The why her? Why me? What will happen next? How will this end? What do I have to learn or do to make this better? Where does the blame land? Why aren't they trying to find the root of the problem and try to fix it from there? Why are they giving her medication that causes what one of her problems is? How can we get any control back? How can there be a future? And every other human thought and emotion went through me. Whenever I would release control to others, I would be so out of balance. So was that the lesson, illusion of control - cleared and released, check.

One of my friend's teachers talked to me. He told me it was all my fault!! Wanted me to go into debt so that he could fix me. And therefore, save my daughter's life. During our video chat at one point, there was a blue line over his entire body. He even pretended it was his Lightsaber. I took a minute and decided not to pay him all this money that very night we spoke. He sent a long text saying my daughter would die because I was not strong enough to do the work on myself. He did apologize the next morning and then slammed me again. To the universe, I sent out thanks for pointing out my imprint that attracts men that want to put me in debt had not been cleared yet. Addressed, released and done, check. Spirit relayed to me that the blue line over this man was Archangel Michael's sword. I started working on myself like never before; I was not afraid of the work. Bring IT!!! I did everything I knew. I listen to Spirit and watched for signs for guidance. I personalize Love Declarations. I watched videos and came up with Project 4 and all that followed. Bottom line my lesson learned was my daughter and all that happens are here to help me remember to live in the moment and find something no matter how small to be grateful for, so that can grow.

I like to find the root of the problem with my patients and work from there. That was not what was happening with my daughter's care. Specialist look at their little set of parameters with no idea it seems that there was more to the body or what a whole body was. What I had tried did not work, I would let them try something. I would let go of ego. I did not care who, what, or how she got better, I just wanted it done yesterday, or last year, or before she was born. Everything they tried did not work for long, even if it did work at all. I was lost.....

A friend of mine, who was watching the hell I was going through handed me a spark to light hope within me once again. For this, I will be forever Grateful!!!! He sent me an email with links to a tv show about Anthony Stephan the founder of Truehope, a lecture by Professor Julia Rucklidge call "What if... Nutrition Could Treat Mental Illness?", and Solgar Formula V VM - 75.

Anthony Stephan had lost his Father - in - Law and wife to mental illness. When 2 of this children were heading down the same path, and regular Medicine was of no help, Anthony hit his knees in Prayer. One day in his church a fellow member walks by and ask about his family. This was an animal nutritionist, he said when the pigs are going crazy we give them more vitamins and minerals, and they get better. So they went to the drug store and made up a mixture to be like the pig supplement. Anthony gave only this to his son. Within 30 days things were looking positive. The supplement also helped Anthony's daughter. For the first time in years, the future was finally looking bright for the Stephans. Truehope said their product does not help everyone. Professor Rucklidge showed scientific research that proved Stephan's case was not just a fluke. Solgar was the brand of Vitamins my friend himself had found and taken to help with depression, gut issues, and other stress-related issues.

Where was the harm in giving a Vitamin Supplement????? It fit right in with; it might help and not hurt why not try?? This made sense to my

Veterinary brain. When I was done researching all these links, I wanted the Vitamins before she was born. My friend brought some over to me. He handed them to me, and I could feel the energy firing up my spine. I went to examine the label to see if valerian was in it or not. I could not read the small print. I took a dose, started talking to my friend, and about 2 minutes later flipped the bottle over and could read the small print. So the debate between daughter and mother continues to this day if these help or not. My last remark to her was, "it makes me feel better when you take them, even if nothing else is improved."

Once I have hope once again, I could hear my guides, they keep saying to me "permeable barriers and inflammation." I interpreted it as leaky gut and things passing through the blood-brain barrier that did not belong which would lead to inflammation. This also made perfect sense to me, but all of her doctors thought I was from another planet. Every free moment I sat at my computer to try to find some help. This just frustrated my daughter, "there you go being Dr. Google, just like what owners do that upsets you." One day a Darling friend sat in my chair in front of my computer, and within minutes she was telling me to give my daughter Colostrum to treat leaky gut. Confirmation, thank you, Universe. One by one, I found Doctors that had figured out this gut-brain connection. I can't tell you the order in which I found them, but they were out there mostly from their own experience or they had watched patients repeatedly improve. Finding others helped me, but still was not helpful for daughter and her doctors.

Her doctors would blow it off, that there is no research. And they had never heard of that, etc.

I did try to get my daughter into one of the ones on the list, but insurance would not cover something that might actually cure anything...

David Perlmutter, MD The Empowering Neurologist, Grain Brain, https://www.drperlmutter.com/

Kelly Brogan, MD Own Your Body. Free your Mind. http://kellybroganmd.com/

Steven Gundry, MD is a cardiologist, heart surgeon, medical researcher, and author. "The Plant Paradox," http://gundrymd.com/

Mark Hyman, MD, Broken Brain, The Ultra Mind Solution, http://drhyman.com/

Amy Myers, MD Get to the root. Learn the tools. Live the Solution. https://www.amymyersmd.com/

Gut and Psychology Syndrome (GAP Syndrome or GAPS) is a condition which establishes a connection between the functions of the digestive system and the brain. This term was created by Dr. Natasha Campbell–McBride, MD, MMedSci (neurology), MMedSci (human nutrition) in 2004 after working with hundreds of children and adults with neurological and psychiatric conditions, such as autistic spectrum disorders, attention deficit hyperactivity disorder (ADHD / ADD), schizophrenia, dyslexia, dyspraxia, depression, obsessive-compulsive disorder, bipolar disorder and other neuropsychological and psychiatric problems. http://www.gaps.me/
Find out more about Dr. Campbell-McBride at www.doctor-natasha.com

During this stressful time, my body was also starting to yell for help. My A1C had raised up, and my Liver values indicated surgery was in my near future. Another friend of mine showed me a video on her phone about "The Gerson Therapy" during one of our long drives to see my daughter. Charlotte Gerson carries on her father's work successfully treating thousands of patients with one of the first alternative cancer therapies. It uses juicing, coffee enemas, and supplements. I had already been juicing and knew how much better I was with it. The next day, I increased my juicing and ordered a coffee enema kit. At first, I was juicing in the morning and doing the coffee enema at night. I detox big time. Then I started juicing and coffee enemas as Spirit, my body, and my schedule allowed. I would not do either one when I had to chiropractically adjust a horse that day. I wanted to be able to bend over safely. In less than three months my liver values were completely healthy, my A1C was down significantly and substantial release of body weight.

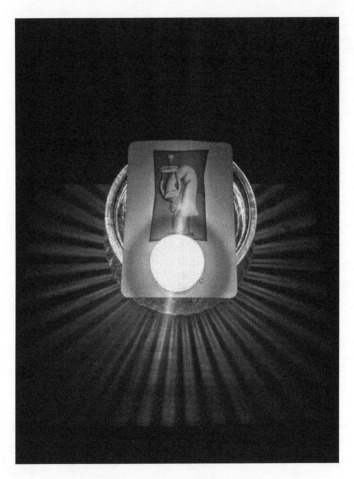

The only time I pulled this card was just
before my first Coffee Enema

Coffee enemas had been listed in the Merck Manual, but have been removed. Not a big money maker for Modern Medicine. As I learned it was started when a "MASH" camp was locked in without supplies. The patients were in extreme pain, and there was coffee on the stove for the surgeons. I don't know if I would have made that connection, but am grateful someone had been inspired. It has a great many uses: detox; drug detox; nicotic detox; gallbladder pumping / clean out; clearing brain fog; etc. Another friend of mine had gone from needing kidney dialysis to normal by doing a coffee enema every other day for six weeks. The coffee needs to be caffeinated and should be organic. My daughter has informed me many times, "No coffee is getting close to that end of the body." More learning lessons: what are you willing to do to get better, I can't make others do what I think may be helpful, and my old favorite you can't help those that don't want help.

I absolutely Loved Anthony William since I picked up his first book *"Medical Medium: Secrets Behind Chronic and Mystery Illness and How to Finally Heal."* Since he was very young, there is a voice just outside of this ear that he can not turn off. The first thing it told him was his Grandmother had lung cancer. I need to be high energy and need to check in to hear my "Spirit". I had lumped all these Mystery Illness together, but never put a name or a cause to them as Anthony has done. I love getting Divine Guidance over scientific research every time. My daughter did test positive to Lymes and Epstein Barr in a transdermal scan, but negative through traditional testing. I had homeopathic bottles made based on the transdermal scan. My daughter would not take it. Whenever I thought about it, I would hold the bottles and dowse all that was needed within these bottles to energetically go into my daughter and me. Just as I had watched Raymon Grace do years before with his supplements.

Reading about what to eat and not eat drove me insane!!! For a while, I just threw my hands up in the air and gave up. I am a single working Mom, her schedule and my schedule can be unbelievable. I was told I would write three books over 20 years ago. My response up to now was, I don't have time to read a book, let alone write one. I totally admit we are both lovers of SAD (Standard American Diet). Our Microbiomes (gut flora) crave and push us to eat all the things not so good for us. I juice and detox, She wants to vomit from the smell. Spirit finally total me to do as I often tell my clients. Do the best you can. Do muscle response testing as often as you can. Pay attention if something causes problems. If it does avoid it if possible, do an Allergy Elimination Treatment, dowse everything you consume, and / or reprogram your body to benefit from it. However, the book that resonates best to my horses and me is *"The Earth Diet: Your Complete Guide to Living Using Earth's Natural Ingredients"* by Liana Werner-Gray.

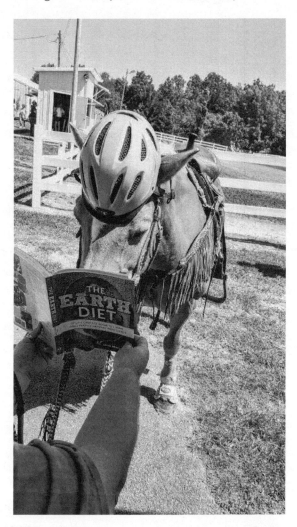

I also truly believe one of the main things that I did not see in all the diet information, is the amount of love in the food. No matter what organic ingredients or over process products my daughter and / or I am putting together for us to consume it has Love in it !!!! The only Love in fast food is from the Microbiome and Corporate America. I feel that is why many are taught to Pray, Bless, dowse, etc. because it adds Love to the food.

The Microbiome is just like Seymore in the Little Shop of Horrors. FEED ME whatever the bacteria is in need of. And there is a craving that often cannot be stopped. You eat what you crave which feeds and grows more of that bacteria. This loop continues until we are gone. This fits right in with you are what you eat. We are just a host for this universe of bacteria within us. As in the Matix do you chose the red or blue pill??? The Microbiome can be weakened by how you are born (c - section), stress, toxins, medications. etc. This is why probiotic are everywhere now yogurt, gummies, food, drinks, etc. The Microbiome can be changed by changing what you consume live through the die-off of old bacteria and regrowth of the new type of bacteria. Another way though maybe not so pleasant is the fecal transplant.

Fecal transplant or as I like to call it, poop soup, can be amazingly effective to a huge number of things including claims of autism, Parkinson, etc.. I have been to lots of lectures on this and keep finding more things it can help. But Modern Medicine does not make much money off of this either. Back in the 1930's, they would do fecal transplant from happy people into clinically sad people, and they would become happy. C. Diff is 100% curable with a fecal transplant. Why it is better to let people die than share poop??? However, I am not probability ever going to get my daughter to do this either. So I pray, dowse, compassion, ho'oponopono, and whatever else I can do for myself and her.

Amy Myers, MD has a practice and online presence that promotes her products that helps control Candida. She claims lots of other symptoms go away once Candida is under control. I believe what she says to be true. I am willing to do anything, within most laws, for my daughter. I have learned that, if I think it will help and buy it, she will not want it and will not take it. Spirit told me to use what I already had here. The next morning Spirit and I came up with another doTERRA Essential Oil Mixture bottle, but this time for Candida. It is very high energy and has helped many living things already. I now carry a roller bottle of this in my pocket to apply to my patients, daughter, and self as often as I can.

I try to be in the moment and listen to what my daughter is saying. As in the video "Heal Yourself; Mind Over Medicine" by Lissa Rankin, M.D. Sometimes she is telling me what she needs to heal or writing her own prescription for health. I am not saying give them everything they want, even though many that see us may often think that is what I do. I follow my heart, Spirit, and Divine Timing to patiently as much as possible, wait and see what comes, because it is already on its way. Sometimes it seems like, to me, she is non stop complaining. In these times I try to remember something from a Matt Kahn video. Do not take personal what is being yelled at you, because they are just telling you what they need deep down to heal. So most of the time I am doing ho'oponopono and / or Moses Code and being so Grateful my daughter is still here with me to be able to have this experience and then repeat the next moment!!!!!!

What doesn't kill you makes you stronger. I cannot stop all the possible "bad" that might come at my daughter and me. I had heard one person talking about crustaceans. Stress is needed for the shell to come off. They then hide while they are vulnerable and increase in size and grow a new shell. If there were no stress, there would be no growth. What we have been through has made us stronger, better able to help those that walk that path with us. This makes me a better Shaman, which means "Wounded Healer."

In this dream, called life, I chose to grow while on this amazing journey. I decided / Universe pushed to share with you just a small burp of what I have learned along the way. Thank you for coming and being my witness. I pray that by sharing some of my Pearl of Wisdom, you hopefully do not have to reinvent the wheel if you find yourself in a similar path.

Blessing of Love, Light, Healing, and Dunamas to you and yours all the way back to Adam or your Source.

PRAYER WARRIOR ON.

AHO.

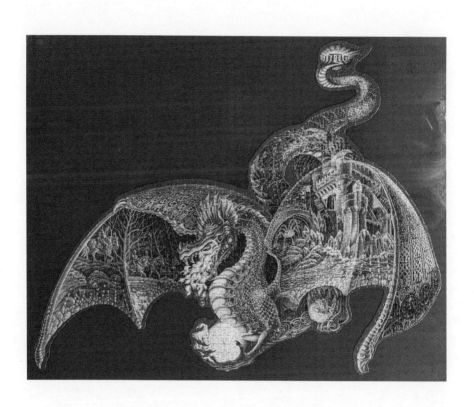

References

Green, Janet, "The Reiki Healing Bible, Transmit healing energy through your hands to achieve deep relaxation, inner peace, and total well-being", Chartwell Book, New York, New York, CR 2012. ISBN 13: 978-0-7858-2964-5

Paul, Ph.D. Nina L., "Reiki for Dummies", Wiley Publishing, Inc, CR 2006, ISBN-10: 0-7645-9907-1.

Morris, M.S., C.A.D.C, Reiki Master Teacher Joyce J., "Reiki Hands That Heal", Weiser Books, Boston, MA/York Beach, ME, CR 1996, ISBN 1-57863-118-1

Stein, Diane, "Essential Reiki, A Complete Guide to An Ancient Healing Art'", Crossing Press, Berkeley/Toronto, CR 1995, ISBN 13: 978-0-89594-736-9, ISBN-10: 0-89594-736-6

Gordon, Richard, "Quantum Touch, The Power To Heal, North Atlantic Books, Berkeley, California, CR 1999. 2022, 2006, ISBN 1-55643-594-0, https://quantumtouch.com/

Grace, Raymon, founder and president of Raymon Grace Foundation, is a dowser, lecture and author of 3 books,"The Future is Yours—Do Something About It", "Techniques That Work For Me" and "Seasons of April." http://www.raymongrace.us/

Grabhorn, Lynn, "Dear God! What's Happening To Us? Halting Eons of Manipulation", Hampton Roads Publishing Company, Inc. Charlottesville, VA CR 2003, ISBN 1-57174-384-7

Haner, Jean, "Clear Home, Clear Heart learn to clear the energy of people & places," Hay House, Inc. Carlsbad, California, New York City, London, Sydney, Johannesburg, Vancouver, New Delhi, CR 2017 ISBN 978-1-4019-5154-2, https://www.jeanhaner.com/

Diamond, Marie, Diamond Dowsing, http://www.mariediamond.com/

Mannix, Edward founder of The Compassion Key ®, https://compassionkey.com/, http://edwardmannix.com/

Twyman, James F., "The Moses Code The Most Powerful Manifestation Tool in the History of the World", Hay House, 2/11/10, ISBN: 9781401917890

Ho'oponopono Course/Certification by Dr. Joe Vitale, Mathew Dixon, Dr. Ihaleakala Hew Len, · http://www.hooponoponocertification.com/.

Virtue, Doreen, "10 Messages Your Angels Want You to Know," Hay House, Inc., Publication Date: 5/2/17, ISBN: 9781401952723

Hale, Mandy, http://thesinglewoman.net/about/

Angelou, Maya was an American poet, singer, memoirist, and civil rights activist. She published seven autobiographies, three books of essays, several books of poetry, and was credited with a list of ... Wikipedia

Rumi, Jalāl ad-Dīn Muhammad Rūmī, also known as Jalāl ad-Dīn Muhammad Balkhī, Mevlânâ/Mawlānā, Mevlevî/Mawlawī, and more popularly simply as Rumi, was a 13th-century Persian Sunni Muslim poet, jurist, Islamic scholar, theologian, and Sufi mystic. Wikipedia

Wiseman, Sara, http://www.sarawiseman.com/

Kahn, Matt, Whatever Arises Love That, http://www.truedivinenature.com/

Openshaw, Robyn, Green Smoothie Girl, https://greensmoothiegirl.com/

Sheldon, Christie Marie, https://christiesheldon.com/

Robbins, Mel, https://melrobbins.com/

Morrissey, Mary, http://www.marymorrissey.com/

Beckwith, Michael, http://www.michaelbernardbeckwith.com/

Demartini, DC John, https://drdemartini.com/

Stec, L. M. Bluehawks, "Indigenous Medicine Wheel Of All People (Four and Eight Spoke)" CR 2008, 2013, ISBN: 978-0-9815815-3-8

Stephan, Anthony, the founder of Truehope, https://www.truehope.com/about/the-truehope-story

Rucklidge, Professor Julia, lecture "What if... Nutrition could treat mental illness?", https://www.youtube.com/watch?v=FrxdoIn6DQQ

Solgar Formula V VM - 75, http://www.solgar.com/SolgarProducts/Formula-VM-75-Tablets.htm

Perlmutter, MD David, The Empowering Neurologist, Grain Brain, https://www.drperlmutter.com/

Brogan, MD Kelly, Own Your Body. Free your Mind. http://kellybroganmd.com/

Gundry, MD Steven is a cardiologist, heart surgeon, medical researcher, and author. "The Plant Paradox", http://gundrymd.com/

Myers, MD Amy, Get to the root. Learn the tools. Live the Solution. https://www.amymyersmd.com/

Hyman, MD Mark, Broken Brain, The Ultra Mind Solution, http://drhyman.com/

Campbell–McBride, MD Natasha, MMedSci (neurology), MMedSci (human nutrition), http://www.doctor-natasha.com/ Gut and Psychology Syndrome (GAP Syndrome or GAPS), http://www.gaps.me/

Gerson, Charlotte, The Gerson Therapy, Gerson Institute. https://gerson.org/gerpress/

William, Anthony was born with the ability to converse with a high-level spirit. Medical Medium, http://www.medicalmedium.com/

Werner-Gray, Liana, "The Earth Diet: Your Complete Guide to Living Using Earth's Natural Ingredients", Hay House, CR 2014, ISBN: 978-1-1-4019-4497-1

Rankin, M.D., Lissa, video "Heal Yourself; Mind Over Medicine," http://lissarankin.com/

Potential Future Books or Services Available

This part was so hard to write because I AM always growing.

It would have been a lot easier to list what I do not do....

- Put needles in horses Ting Points by hand.
- Major or Orthopedic surgery and fracture repair.
- Traditional Medical Treatment of Diabetes, Cushings, Addison, etc.
- Eat Marcinho Cherries or Black Liquorice.
- Drink Root Beer or any other Beer.

THE BOOK OF FRANK

Frank looks like regular Orange male short hair tiger striped domestic shorthair feline. However, that is about where the similarity to regular cats very. I often tell clients he is just walking around in a cat body. He knows where the problem is in humans and animals. He calms almost everything that comes to the clinic. He performed tons of yoga moves to get a yoga instructor's attention. He has had empathic spasms with other animals during their treatments. Some clients call him Dr. Frank.

He is a Healing Master, my teacher, my helper, my familiar and so much more....

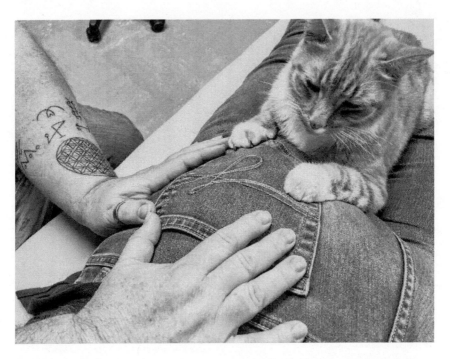

HALO BASSET THE HERO AND WORLD CHANGER

Halo is a basset hound who told me on our first visit as a 6-week old puppy that she was in her 2nd reincarnation during my daughter's life, her name was Halo, and she was back for my daughter. She had been a Great Dane, Taffy, who was old when my daughter was born. Then she was a special kitten, that carrier the Great Dane energy. It would make me laugh watching all the unusual reactions in man and beast to this kitten. Halo made significant positive changes to my home even before she was able to come home to stay. For many years it may seem like she was just a regular beloved pet. When my daughter was in need Halo's God-given abilities are nothing short of Miracle after Miracle after Miracle.

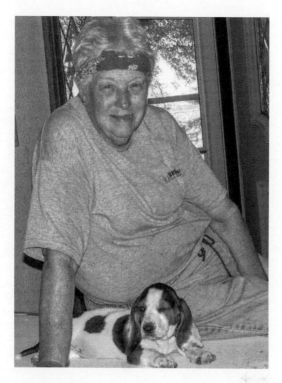

Mommers and Baby Halo getting new pet friendly flooring

AWESOMENESS CUBED HOLISTIC EMERGENCY KITS AND ACUPRESSURE POINTS

List of natural products and acupressure points for general use or an emergency. Did you know there is an Acupressure / Acupuncture point that can restart breathing and the heart? It is GV 26, but I like to call it the Reset Button. It can be used any time, but especially if shock, collapse, and seizures. I think everyone should be empowered to know it and possibly save a life.....

It is the midline point of the upper lip gum margin. If not dire, pressure can be applied to the outside of the skin. If no response, then going under the lip. If cardiac and / or respiratory failure and a needle is available, henpeck to the bone. For most things put your finger under the nose. For birds, I have had people apply pressure just above the beak. If worried about your finger's safety, you can use a retracted pen or mechanical pencil.

So if you can't figure out where the Reset Button is, mentally draw a mustache on whatever it is that is in need of help. Then this magical point is in the center of the mustache. Except on birds, try just above the beck in the center.

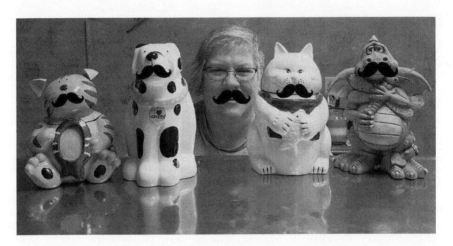

I love to do demonstrations of these points, especially for kids. I cover points that help stop bleeding, GI issues, breathing issues, pain, and seizures. I first show them where the points are on humans. Halo Basset gets placed on a table, and everybody has to feel each point on her. Just another example of her World Changing ways.

AWESOMENESS CUBED SNELL HEALING HANDS METHODS

I am always learning, growing and combining techniques. I have been inspired and lead by Spirit while working on man and beast. I often spend an hour during a session. The patient is usually entirely different in so many ways in that treatment. I have many animals cannot walk in and can walk either after first or couple treatments. I have also helped so many people with a bad joint that needed "surgery". They often go from bad to normal in sometimes in as little as a couple minutes to a session. Of course, perfect results are not guaranteed, but be open to the possibility.

AWESOMENESS CUBED STICK HEALING METHOD

I have been learning, adding, and growing to use a stick as an extension of my hands. I send energy down the stick to release so many unneeded things and so much more. I use it to help the horse adjust its own back. With the stick putting me at a much safer distance.....
I am also adapting these stick moves for aggressive dogs and cats.

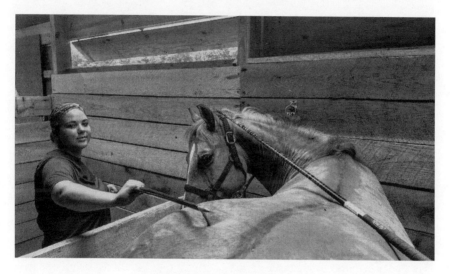

Megan Lyons and Newt

AWESOMENESS CUBED VERTEBRAL STACKING

When a vertebra falls forwards, there is no muscle combination that can self-correct this problem. The typical pushdown chiropractic movement of the spine also does not release this forward vertebra. As I do, combining learned and Spirit-inspired come up with a moving technique to correct these forward vertebrae. When all vertebra is inline, so many awesomeness things happen to improve self-healing and decrease pain.

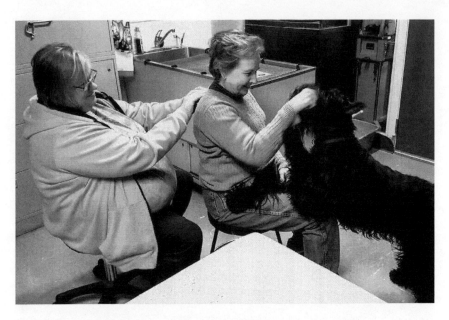

AWESOMENESS CUBED BACK TO WALKING

The list is very long of animals that had no hope of walking anywhere else and returned to normal or at least greatly improved...

This filly is just one example. Three times a backhoe was called because she could not get up and then canceled. Will she race or not is yet to be determined. But alive, joyful, and running she is.

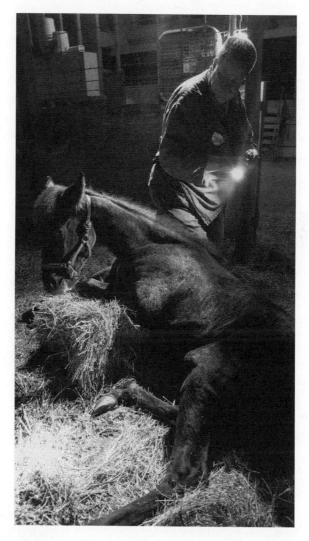

ACCESS BARS

I run bars on my patients to help release pass issues quickly and painlessly. Spirit has had me combine them with various acupuncture points to assist in this process. This is great for rescued animals or anyone with past trauma. I have now started running bars on animals before the end of life with the intent to help release everything but the lessons and the love. To go to the Rainbows the best they can be and hopeful not reincarnate with extra unwanted baggage.

When I run horse's bars, a vortex opens up to vacuum away all that is discharged. I now have to give owners a warning, that this may also affect them if the connection between them is secure. Many owners get dizzy with some having to lay down on the ground. One owner entirely left their body. With one hand I was trying to keep this horse pictured below off of the owner. With my other hand I was assisting the limp body while it was sliding down the stall wall then landed on the ground. On the owners return to this dimension, they relayed their travels and took a little time to process and fully reconnect.

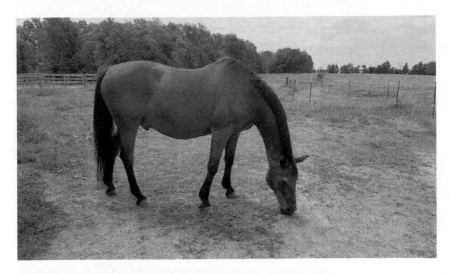

AWESOMENESS CUBED BODY TWISTER

I came up with this name because that is what it seems like to me. During a session, my guides will say right hand here, left hand there, right foot on their right foot, and left foot on their left foot or where ever. I feel blocked pathways open up.

This Body Twister can produce amazing unexpected things. Once a Mother and High School aged rapidly growing son came in together for a session for him. Mom was always telling him to sit up straight. Later they were telling me he was failing PE because he could not bend over far enough, pictured below. When I asked Spirit what I could do to help him we started the Twister game. I would hold that position, the boy would unwinded until he was on the ground. He would get up, test how far he could bend over, and we would do it again. After 3 or 5 times he could stand on his fingers. Later that evening I got the memo from Spirit, that he could not sit up straight was the same reason as the legs. His bones had grown faster than his tendons had stretched. I relayed to Mom and I did Body Twister on the top half of him the next time. He can sit up straight after Vertebral stacking and Body Twister. Now whenever he feels he cannot bend or move they are back for another visit. He is now passing PE, back to playing Football, and Dr. Frank helped!

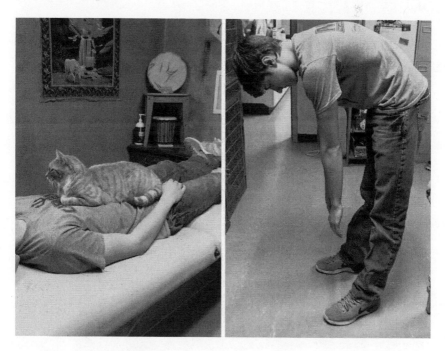

LASER THERAPY

Doreen Virtue claims healing begins or happens from LOVE and LIGHT. We already had the LOVE. The laser adds exponential strength to the LIGHT. Spirit has inspired me to use the laser in so many unconventional ways. When I first started combining Laser with other forms of therapy is when people started falling over or passing out in the exam room, while the pet would be just fine. It took me a little while to figure out that it was the healing vortex spinning faster that was the culprit.

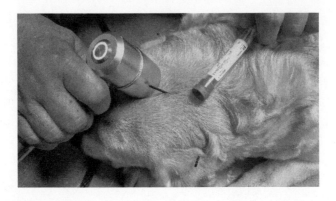

ACUPUNCTURE

I am a Certified Veterinary Acupuncturist. With this training, I feel I understand, treat and can explain to others where the root of the problem lies. It often brings a lot of seemingly unrelated issues a reason to be going on together. The dog pictured above has black acupuncture needles.

VETERINARY ORTHOPEDIC MANIPULATION (VOM)

VOM was my first class for adjusting animals. I have learned, been inspired, and added tons of things to my adjusting process.

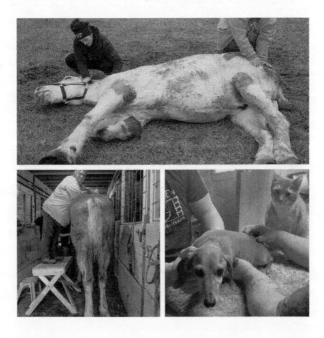

ALLERGY ELIMINATION

A painless process to potentially permanently remove allergies from a living being. Spirit has added many extra things to the initial Veterinary Nambudripad's Allergy Elimination Technique (NAET) treatment.

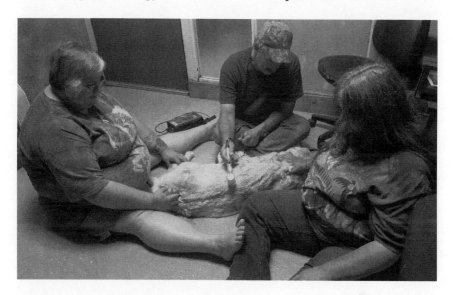

ANIMAL COMMUNICATION

I went to a weekend class on animal communication shortly after my daughter was born. The first words I ever heard a dog speak to me will always make me laugh. He begged me to tell his mother to turn off the new (age) music because it was depressing the h*** out of him.

I often ask how did this trauma happen? I then see a picture of the scene of the incident usually from the animal's point of view and often feel the change.

EMPATHIC ABILITY

I often can feel others pain. I grew tired of feeling everyone's pain. So I asked to move on to knowing about the pain and how to fix it. I frequently "see" or "hear" what needs to be done.

CHANNEL

I can share or give full control of my body over to my guides. While I am doing Healing work on others sometimes I will share control to allow the needed healing to come through.

AWESOMENESS CUBED PERSONAL DILUTION BOTTLES

Tons of bottles are made at Sycamore Animal Hospital for each individual patient. Bottles that can be given orally can contain Homotoxicolity, Homeopathics, Bach Flowers, Willard Water, and possibly Chinese Herbal Formulas. Bottles to be used topically contain doTERRA Essential Oils and other things. A Zyto Compass for doTERRA oils is frequently used to get a baseline of what the patient needs, so all of these tested for are included in the Personal Dilution Bottle. There is no harm to run the scan and a surrogate is used for animal testing. I feel by doing this we are not missing something that might be needed more so on an emotional level.

I am a doTERRA Essential Oil consultant, www.mydoterra.com/sandrasnell. DoTERRA is my oil of choice because I can feel the energy. Every single doTerra bottle I have touched is vibrating with amazing energy. I choose to raise vibration, rather than fight. Within a month of using doTERRA Essential Oils in my home and clinic, I received my Aha moment. The Essential Oils work far better than the herbs because of several things. First, they are easy to get them into the patient. I had given up on getting herbs into a cat. With the oils, you can put them on topically or if that's a problem diffuse them. But no one that I know of has stopped breathing the diffused oil. Though, my smart Orange Healing Cats, Frank and Jophiel, would knock over the diffuser placed in front of their cage when they had a head cold. Most importantly the Essential Oil contains the Life Force Energy of the plant, where the herb is from the old dried up carcass...

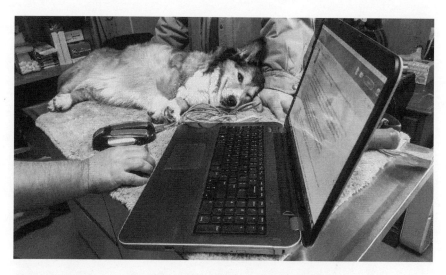

PREVENT OR STOP PROGRESSION OF HIP DYSPLASIA

When I took VOM class, the instructor had done a test with a litter of puppies. He said if the puppies got reads T11 - L 2 and they were cleared out they would not get hip dysplasia. If the reads were not treated these puppies did get hip dysplasia. I have seen this in action so many times. I have expanded my beliefs that if the root of all evil is cleared out then so many problems will be prevented, progression slowed or stopped including hip dysplasia, back, and knee problems.

SEIZURES 101

In Chineses Medicine almost all seizures stims from Liver imbalance. In Western Medicine, all medications that I am aware of for seizure causes Liver Damage. DO NOT stop the current medications, because that could make things worst. Do things to help the liver. Know the acupressure points to help stop seizures and the reset button.

Press Governing Vessel (GV) 20 and both Gallbladder (GB) 20 to help stop and possible prevent seizures. I call it the Volcin Mind Lock for seizures, pictured below. Place your index finger of you dominate hand on the highest boney point on the back of the dog or cat's skull. Put your thumb and ring finger together. Lay them down at dorsal middle line. Open them up along the back of the skull. Stop when they fall into big holes behind the ears. Apply as much pressure as you for as long as allowed. If this is not helping you can also press the Reset Button, GV - 26, pictured above with Emergency Acupressure Points. This point is midline just under the nose. The upper lip can be lifted the point is then midline at the lip / gum margin. For pressure at this point use fingernail or retracted pen. If cardiac or respiratory arrest and a needle is available hen peck this point to hit bone, there will be some bleeding with this.

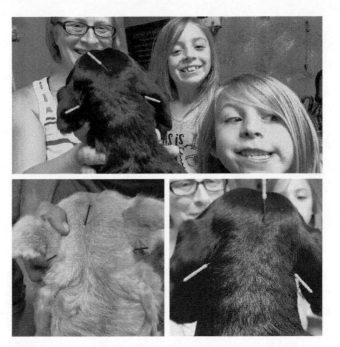

CANCER

I am getting more and more patients that have been given up on by regular medical ways. I never say I can heal this problem... Often I have helped others that were worse off. I believe if it might help and not hurt, why not try??? Even if it does not work, at least there is some emotional relief that everything had been tried...

I help bring the body back into balance to promote self-healing. I relay the messages I am given from Spirit to help. Tools to help antiangiogenesis, decrease carbohydrates, and so much more. Now with adding Ho'oponopono many masses melt in my hands often with Frank's help. Be open to the possibility of spontaneous healing!!!!

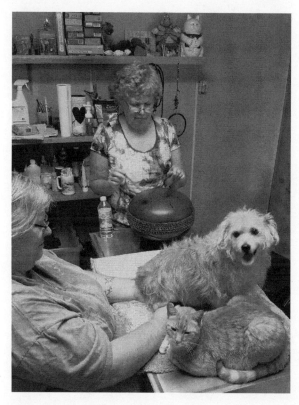

COMBINATION THERAPY and MICKEY LOVES IT!

AWESOMENESS CUBED CIRCLE OF LIFE GUIDED MEDITATION

I have been inspired to put many learned Native American Songs and some Channeled Songs together in a way to help either during an Energy Session or on it own.

AWESOMENESS CUBED MERKABA RIDES

I have been inspired to use people's own energy center as their personal time machine.

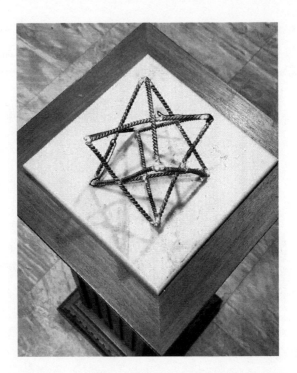

AWESOMENESS CUBED PAST LIFE DEATHS

One of my gifts that started after my Reiki II attunement was to be able to see / feel how someone has died before.

AWESOMENESS CUBED SOUL RETRIEVAL

I have had my Soul Retrieval done by a Shaman. I have performed many for others.

AWESOMENESS CUBED MUSIC THERAPY

I use vocal and a very wide variety of instruments and other noise makers to raise the vibration. I love to sing Tuning, channeled healing songs, and Amazing Grace. Spirit has given me a whole new verse to Amazing Grace. Often the sound that is heard is bigger than me.

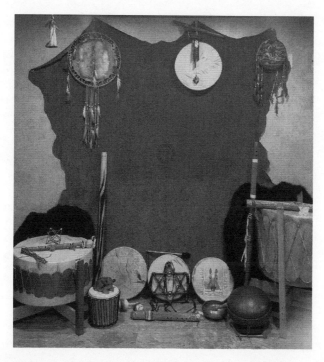

AWESOMENESS CUBED HOUSE / BUSINESS BLESSINGS

Walk through in person or Distance. Moving into a haunted house / property has given me first hand experience. And enough stories for its own book.

AWESOMENESS CUBED TRANSITION / TRANSCENDENCE ASSISTANCE

I have helped many families find peace after a loved one has passed. I have also worked with suicide victims' spirit and survivors to embrace the Light and get answers that are so desperately needed.

I do offer euthanasia, but of course, I do not stop with the physical body I make sure the soul goes to get healed...

I frequently do Energy Healing Sessions with people holding their beloved pet.

AWESOMENESS CUBED TEACHING

I love to teach those that are open and willing. I have released the fear that my students will take business away from me. There are more things needing / wanting my help then I can provide. If my teaching can be used to help others in need, I am truly grateful. I am willing to let go of ego to throw the stone in a new direction for the ripples to grow with or without me. However, I am not the teacher to give all the answers, because learning to ask yourself / your own guides is one of the hardest lessons.

I have helped one very talented pre vet student who shadowed me, get accepted into OSU Vet School on her first attempt. That was 4 years ago and her letter of recommendation was about 3 pages long. Within that letter I had described how Vicky Johnson had become more like family.

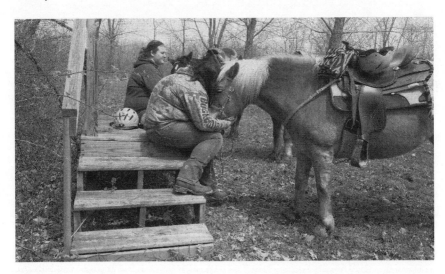

Megan Lyon's is my second pre vet student shadow. She is in this book frequently and she even is the photographer of the cover picture. Megan and the first student are so very talented with amazing Gifts to be shared with the world. This writing thing might be getting a little easier for me. I just submitted Megan's recommendation photo documentary letter and it was 19 pages long. I even used Mosses Code,

Ho'oponopono, and Expanded Release within the letter. Some of it is shared here.

I am Sandra M Snell, DVM, CVA, PSc. D, Reiki Master, Shaman Practitioner, I am. I am about to publish my first book, which is very exciting and hard to believe. I hardly have time to read a book, let alone write one. **I absolutely LOVE Megan Lyons** *and will miss her greatly as she moves forward on her path! She is already a HEALER, but just like me she has an unquenchable thirst for knowledge. She dreams to be a Veterinarian. For all the animals she will help, I hope Dr. Megan Lyons happens as soon as possible.*

I am sorry *your job is hard trying to shift through all of the applications. There is even some concern that your focus may not be on the best criteria.*

Megan Lyon's Essential Oil Cheat Sheet of my favorite oils for different medical uses.

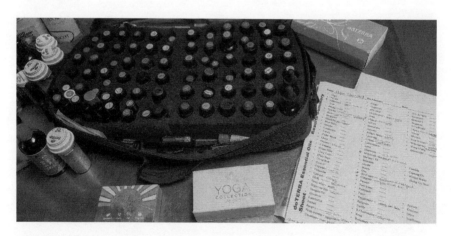

Megan Lyons is smart and determined. Even with a blood clot in her head and being out at least a week of school she ended that session with a 3.8 GPA. This dog had a small wound of its neck, that would bleed non stop in the middle of the night. So I thought to put the e collar on like a hula skirt. Megan was the one to figure out how to keep it on that way. This worked like a charm, the hind legs could not reach the neck and it healed quickly without any more middle of the night emergencies.

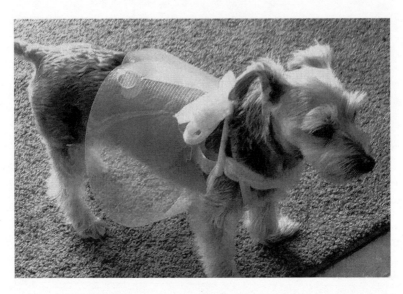

Megan Loves Helping and Learning New things. Clifford the Big Red Dog with Cancer receiving Acupuncture. "Mom" has to take pictures to share with others. My Healing Cats Frank and Jophiel always there to help. With Ho'oponopono Clifford's masses left at the surgical incision site shrink in minutes.

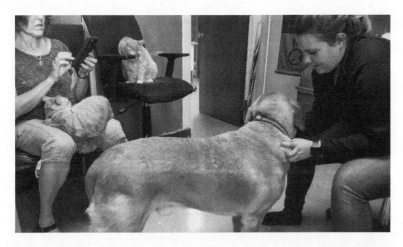

Megan and my daughter, working on my cat Jophiel who had a UTI. I sat and watched quietly as the client while they worked on him. In one hour they did Energy Healing, Access Bars, Cranial Sacral, Quantum Touch, Acupressure, my version of Nambudripad Allergy Elimination Technique, Chiropractic/ Vertebral Stacking, Laser and Essential Oil Therapy on him.

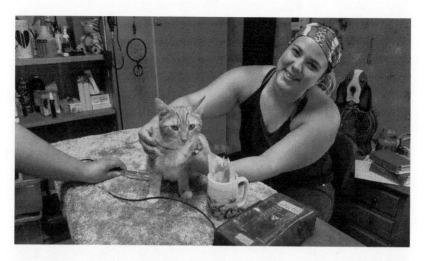

Megan Lyons can be Strong like a Beast when needed. One day I had her play me, and Adjust Coral's haflinger, Chick from start to finish. She proclaimed it is not easy to be Dr. Snell at the end of my video. Chick was not so willing to be picked up and thrown sideways to release the I-S joint and adjust her stifle. However Megan got the job done... After the horse tossing my favorite part is when they look back at you with "What army just picked me up??". Then the lick chews starts up when the job is done right.

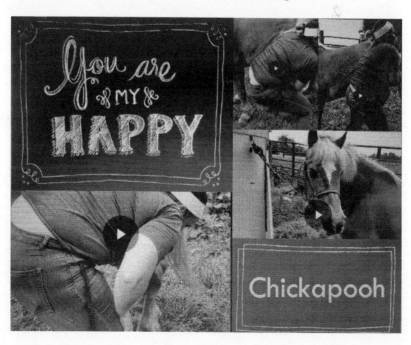

Zeus was non stop yawning during treatment just after huge adjustments in lower neck and brachial plexus. Yawning is often energetic releases. His Mom has certainly never seen him yawn so much at once. Not all yawns were recorded. We used a lot of my new techniques on him which he appreciated immensely. Zeus has not always been the safest horse to adjust in the past. This time with the new things he was safe enough to help teach Megan Lyons...

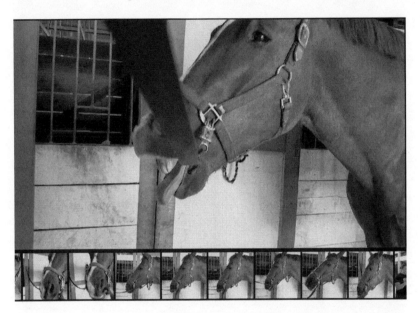

When Zeus was done yawning about 20 times he walked up to Megan to give Thanks.

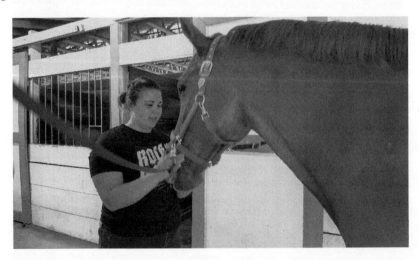

Megan and I worked on Newt during one of our road trips. We were working very well together in a beautiful safe place without time pressure. Megan and I can both shoot healing energy down our cattle show sticks which puts us at a much safer distance. Many new moves were created that day with much laughter in the process. This picture of Megan Lyons from that visit will be in my book under the Awesomeness Cubed Stick Healing Method. Newt's body and pelvis is unwinding.

Please forgive me, *for taking up so much of your time. But I want you to be able to see what a GIFT Megan Lyons is to the World, even if I may be considered outside of the box.*

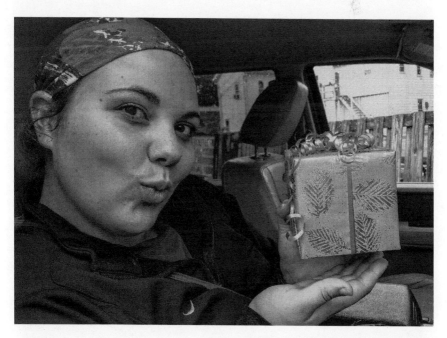

Thank you. *We will be waiting to hear happy news. I release everything but the lessons and the LOVE. I Believe in Miracles. I Believe in You. I Believe in Me. I Believe in Us. I Believe in We. I Believe in the Creator's LOVE and Prosperity. God Bless You and Me.*

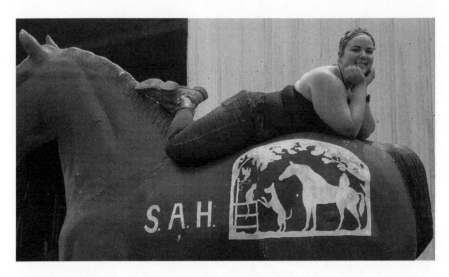

Chynna Rose is a High School Student with dreams of becoming an Animal Massage Therapist and Animal Chiropractor. She is here at Sycamore Animal Hospital through a program of Goodwill Industries. I feel her passion is connected to photograph and artistic things. We have had the best time together creating a lot of the pictures in this book. Thank you Chynna. Please follow your heart to your brightest future possible while remembering your current favorite, always be humble and kind...

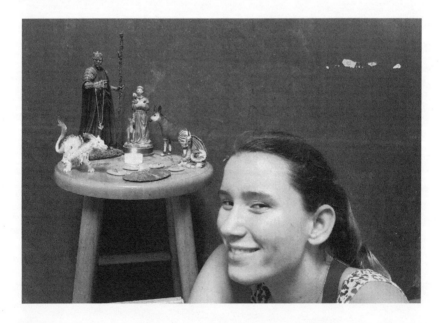

AWESOMENESS CUBED "PIXIE' DUSTING

As the finishing touches are done to this book, Spirit has been giving me one step at a time to a new process using a clay dust that is having the most amazing results on man and beast.....

I PRAY YOU ARE NOW OPEN TO

ENDLESS POSSIBILITIES....

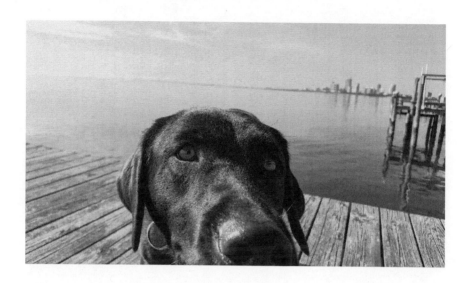

THE END...

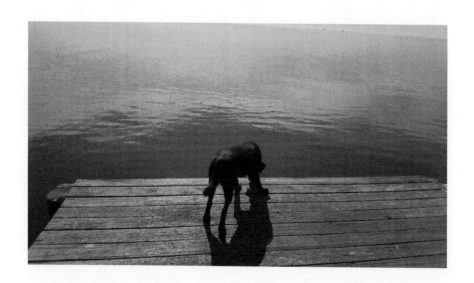

OR IS IT JUST A NEW BEGINNING???

About the Author

Sandra M Snell, DVM, CVA, PSc. D, Reiki Master Teacher, Shaman Practitioner was born with a love of animals that is imprinted into her DNA as much as any other neuropeptide. 4th generation Floridian, she was born and raised in a large city. She was able to manifest her first horse by age 12 by reading the horses for sale in the Sunday paper classified ads to her parents every week. Sandra has not been without at least one horse since then. In 1984 an A.A. degree was received on a full 2 year scholarship for graduating within the top 5% at High School. At the University of Florida she received BS in Animal Science in 1986 and DVM from their College of Veterinary Medicine in 1992. In between the two degrees, she lived and worked at Quail Roost Farm a Thoroughbred Farm in Ocala, Florida.

Sandra's Soul has the need to help loved ones. So she is addicted to learning ways and things that could help in the Healing process of man and beast. She started numerous holistic training all over the US in 1994 including Bach Flowers, NAET, homeopathy, herbs, essential oils, Reiki, Shaman (Native American Medicine Men/Women), Compassion Key, Ho'oponopono, chiropractic, and acupuncture. Sandra became a Certified Veterinary Acupuncturist from the Chi Institute, Redick, FL in 2001. She became a Reiki Master on 4/7/07 and Medicine

Wheel Reiki Master 11/2012. Sandra was Ordained as a Minister of the Universal Life Church 10/2/09. The Pastoral Medical Association on this 25th day of September in the Year of our Lord Two Thousand and Fifteen; hereby Consecrates and Confers Ministerial License of Doctor of Pastoral Science to Dr. Sandra M Snell, PSc. D. This learning and helping have been a passion that has no end.

Sandra's path took a sharp northern turn in 1/1994 to land her in Ohio from south Florida. A week after closing on the house the belongings arrived and were piled into what is now the Clinic. The very next day, a blizzard came in and hit us with a negative 27-degree wind chill. That was toughed out / faced head-on just like every other obstacle. This also demonstrates perfect timing, because if the furniture were still on the truck with negative temperatures, the truck would have been South bond with everything. Sycamore Animal Hospital was open a year later. This has become HOME with hundreds of friends that have become FAMILY.

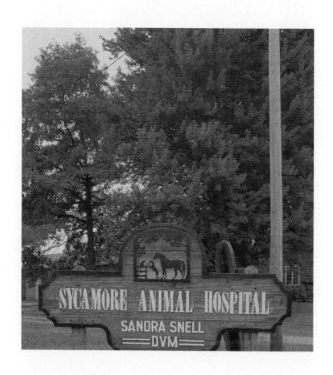

I'LL LEAVE MY LIGHT ON

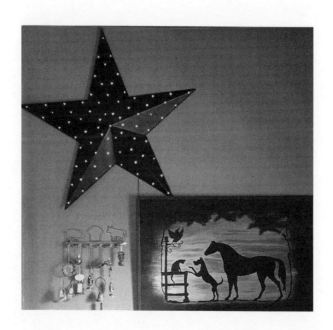

Printed and bound by PG in the USA

USA2019PGIL